I0485828

S. Hrg. 113–680

OVERMEDICATION: PROBLEMS AND SOLUTIONS

HEARING

BEFORE THE

COMMITTEE ON VETERANS' AFFAIRS UNITED STATES SENATE

ONE HUNDRED THIRTEENTH CONGRESS

SECOND SESSION

APRIL 30, 2014

Printed for the use of the Committee on Veterans' Affairs

Available via the World Wide Web: http://www.fdsys.gov

U.S. GOVERNMENT PUBLISHING OFFICE

88–308 PDF   WASHINGTON : 2015

For sale by the Superintendent of Documents, U.S. Government Publishing Office
Internet: bookstore.gpo.gov   Phone: toll free (866) 512–1800; DC area (202) 512–1800
Fax: (202) 512–2104   Mail: Stop IDCC, Washington, DC 20402–0001

COMMITTEE ON VETERANS' AFFAIRS

BERNARD SANDERS, (I) Vermont, *Chairman*

JOHN D. ROCKEFELLER IV, West Virginia
PATTY MURRAY, Washington
SHERROD BROWN, Ohio
JON TESTER, Montana
MARK BEGICH, Alaska
RICHARD BLUMENTHAL, Connecticut
MAZIE HIRONO, Hawaii

RICHARD BURR, North Carolina, *Ranking Member*
JOHNNY ISAKSON, Georgia
MIKE JOHANNS, Nebraska
JERRY MORAN, Kansas
JOHN BOOZMAN, Arkansas
DEAN HELLER, Nevada

STEVE ROBERTSON, *Staff Director*
LUPE WISSEL, *Republican Staff Director*

(II)

CONTENTS

OVERMEDICATION: PROBLEMS AND SOLUTIONS

WEDNESDAY, APRIL 30, 2014

U.S. SENATE,
COMMITTEE ON VETERANS' AFFAIRS,
Washington, DC.

The Committee met, pursuant to notice, at 10:05 a.m., in room 418, Russell Senate Office Building, Hon. Bernard Sanders, Chairman of the Committee, presiding.

Senators present: Senators Sanders, Rockefeller, Begich, Blumenthal, Burr and Isakson.

OPENING STATEMENT OF HON. BERNARD SANDERS, CHAIRMAN, U.S. SENATOR FROM VERMONT

Chairman SANDERS. Let us get to work. Let me thank our panelists for being with us for a really important discussion about a significant issue.

Within the veterans' community—and in fact, throughout our Nation both in the public sector and the private sector—we face a very serious problem of overmedication.

The result of that overmedication is significant numbers of people treated in the Department of Defense facilities, VA facilities, and in the private sector become dependent upon those medications intended to help them and ease their pain. Pain is a huge problem in the country and how we treat that pain in the most effective way is really what we are discussing today.

Some people who are treated with a whole lot of medication become addicted, and I think we all know what happens when people become addicted, in the worst cases some may end up losing their lives due to overdoses. In my State and throughout this country, this is a huge problem.

This is a major issue that has been discussed on this Committee during the last year, and we are so glad we have such a distinguished panel with us today to help us examine this problem.

But, before we get to this issue at hand, I did want to say a very brief word about another issue that has attracted a lot of attention in this country, and that is the developing situation at the VA medical center in Phoenix.

As I think everyone in this room knows, some very, very serious allegations have been made regarding delays in health care access and, as a result, the possible deaths of veterans. I just want to make it very very clear that I take and this Committee takes these allegations extremely seriously; and we are going to do everything we can to get to the bottom of this story and get to the truth.

(1)

Yesterday I spoke to the VA's acting inspector general, Richard Griffin. There is a thorough investigation being conducted by the VA IG in Phoenix and I have been assured by Mr. Griffin that he has the resources he needs to thoroughly investigate that situation.

I expect that the inspector general's office will conduct its investigation thoroughly and provide this Committee with an objective analysis of these very serious allegations. And as I indicated the other day, it is my intention to hold a hearing on this issue once the inspector general's inquiry is complete.

I want to make two brief points on this issue. First, we will get to the bottom of what has happened in Phoenix. We will reach conclusions based on an objective investigation of the facts, not TV reports but an objective investigation of the facts.

Second, we should not let these allegations impugn the excellent work done throughout this country by hundreds of thousands of VA doctors, nurses, administrators, and staff at all levels, many of whom are veterans themselves or are closely related to veterans.

I have been all over this country. I just came back from the VA facility in Minneapolis, MN, and my assessment is that we have some great people there doing great work.

Additionally, a recent survey by the American Consumer Satisfaction Index, an independent consumer service survey, pointed out patient satisfaction is incredibly high within VA—higher, perhaps, than the private sector. And I can tell you in Vermont—and I think this story is true all over this country—that when veterans walk into the VA, they feel very good about the quality of care they get.

And I do not want anything that is happening or may have happened in Phoenix to impugn the very good work done by people throughout this country.

Getting back to the issue at hand, as a Nation, we must remember that for many veterans, chronic pain is a part of their daily life. According to VA data, the most common diagnosis among post-9/11 veterans is musculoskeletal ailments, including joint, neck, and back disorders. Chronic pain is a common symptom of this cluster of conditions.

VA research demonstrates greater than 50 percent of male veterans using VA primary care report instances of chronic pain and the prevalence of chronic pain may be even higher among women veterans.

Therefore, options for managing chronic pain among our veteran population are paramount to improving quality-of-life and re-integration.

Additionally, PTSD, along with other mental health diagnoses, such as depression and anxiety, are frequently diagnosed among our veterans. According to the most recent data from VA, more than 55 percent of our post-9/11 veterans have been diagnosed with some type of mental health disorder.

Just as with chronic pain, it is critical these veterans receive the treatment they need and deserve. Oftentimes, opioids are used to treat both chronic pain and certain mental health disorders. While opioids can be quite effective in treating these conditions, they also come with significant risk which is what we are going to be discussing today.

Therefore, it is critical that these medications are prescribed to the right patients, with careful monitoring and a clear understanding of proper usage.

I would point out that Senator John Boozman of Arkansas has been one of those Senators here who has raised this issue and I think, as we all know, John has been in the hospital with a heart issue. I think I speak for the whole Committee in wishing him the very best of luck and returning to us as soon as possible.

Senator Burr.

STATEMENT OF HON. RICHARD BURR, RANKING MEMBER, U.S. SENATOR FROM NORTH CAROLINA

Senator BURR. Well, thank you, Mr. Chairman, and let me report for my colleagues that Senator Boozman is home. He did not have a heart attack. He had a problem with his aorta. It was not an aneurism. It was a genetic flap that had he not caught it and had they not been able to do a surgical graft on his aorta, he would not have survived like many Americans.

But the report is good. He is home. He will be back with us hopefully soon with a few synthetic parts but I think that by all accounts those synthetic parts work every bit as good as the original.

Mr. Chairman, thank you for this hearing and, as important, thank you to our witnesses for being here.

Since the Chairman has talked about Phoenix, let me just say this. This is not the first issue on quality of care that faces the department, and one veteran death related to delays in care is one too many.

I strongly believe that this Committee needs to hold aggressive oversight hearings into these issues that the department continues to struggle with, including long wait times for specialty care appointments, the misuse of wait lists, and the issues documented in the health care inspections conducted by the inspector general which, by my count, is now over 50 since January 2013.

Even with all of these issues being publicly reported or included in the reports by the IG, this Committee has yet to hold a single oversight hearing on the quality of care veterans are receiving at the VA facilities.

Mr. Chairman, I would fully support and urge you to hold those hearings.

I say as it relates to Phoenix, I think the Chairman is right. Let us get as many of the facts as we can and not rely on what is publicly printed.

But again, I point to the IG investigations from the past and suggest that it is the responsibility of this Committee to respond to some of the problems and to work with the VA, Dr. Petzel, as a partner. And I have never seen the agency shy away from trying to solve those quality of care issues.

Now, turning to today's subject matter, the United States is facing an epidemic of prescription drug abuse. That is why it is important that we are here today to conduct oversight over the care of veterans who have chronic pain. It is critical that we ensure that VA is taking the necessary steps to address the overuse of certain medications and the potential risk of misuse and dual prescriptions.

It has been estimated that as many as 50 percent of male veterans and as high as 75 percent of female veterans—OEF and OIF veterans—struggle with pain.

The prevalence of chronic pain will likely increase as more servicemembers transition into the VA system. These numbers demonstrate the need for VA to provide quality pain management services to ensure veterans with chronic pain are able to live productive and healthy lives.

According to the Centers for Investigative Reporting, between 2001 and 2012 the number of VA prescriptions within four opiate categories—including hydrocodone, oxycodone, methadone, and morphine—surged 270 percent. Additionally, during 2012, VA providers wrote more than 6.5 million prescriptions within those opiate categories.

I found these numbers alarming, in combination with recent media reports that describe veterans with known and documented drug addictions who were still being prescribed these types of medications.

I would just like to highlight a couple of stories. A veteran with PTSD who self-medicated using oxycodone and heroin who later struggled to become clean and sober, who is still struggling with PTSD and his addiction, now faces a new battle with the VA system which continues to prescribe him opiates even though his electronic health record documents his addiction and the subsequent detox provided by VA.

Another veteran, while still on active duty, says he was injecting himself with an anti-inflammatory drug prescribed by military doctors. When he was treated by VA, they only responded to his pain by, ''loading him up on narcotics.'' This veteran goes on to make the following statement, ''There were better options to treat my pain, and those were not presented to me. The priority was treating me the fastest, seemingly least expensive way, and it was the most detrimental.''

Now, I am not sure that this is the patient-centered or veteran-centric care that we constantly hear VA describing. Even in today's testimony from the Department we will hear, ''care is increasingly personalized, proactive and patient driven.''

If these stories reflect what VA believes is personalized, proactive, and patient driven, we have more problems to address than just the quality of care and long wait times.

When it comes to the care we are providing to those who have sacrificed so much for our Nation, we cannot afford to get it wrong. This Committee needs to hold VA accountable to ensure they are providing world-class care.

Right now, with the media reports and even VA's own research, I am not sure we are. Today VA will describe their policies, directives, and initiatives to ensure opiate therapies are prescribed to veterans in a safe manner. It is our obligation to hold VA accountable and to ensure that they are providing the highest standard of care to those who are already in the system.

Mr. Chairman, I thank you for calling this hearing. I look forward to the witnesses' testimony which will enlighten us and the opportunity to follow up with questions.

Chairman SANDERS. Senator Burr, thank you very much.

Senator Blumenthal.

STATEMENT OF HON. RICHARD BLUMENTHAL, U.S. SENATOR FROM CONNECTICUT

Senator BLUMENTAL. Thank you, Mr. Chairman.

I want to thank our witnesses for being here and for your dedicated and hard work to the service of our veterans and our Nation; and thank you, Mr. Chairman and Ranking Member Burr for your comments.

I want to join in expressing my very strong alarm about the reports from Arizona. If true, these reports indicate not only a betrayal of trust but also, very bluntly, violation of our criminal laws in shredding documents and obfuscating evidence that is important to protect the public trust.

So, I hope that the inspector general will complete his report as quickly as possible to restore that trust and confidence in the integrity of our system.

I want place in the record, Mr. Chairman, if I may, a request that we be informed as to what the time table is for completing that investigation because I very much share the Chairman's concern that this Committee has a obligation separately and independently of the inspector general, which has been articulated by the ranking member as well, that we uncover whatever the facts are here and make sure that we fulfill our responsibility. And I believe that if the inspector general's investigation lags that we should proceed independently.

I agree that we should make use of the inspector general's investigation if it proceeds promptly but I think that we should require some kind of preliminary report to us as to what the claims are and what the preliminary findings are because the reports about a secret waiting list, and about neglect of care, and about disregard of the responsibility to provide that care are beyond alarming. They are truly angering.

I want to also express my interest and concern about the subject matter of this investigation. I have seen in Connecticut, as we have around the country, an epidemic of overuse and abuse of these powerful pain killers and other prescription drugs. They are not only deeply concerning themselves, but they are potentially a gateway to other abuse such as heroin.

We have seen in Connecticut and Vermont as well, Mr. Chairman, how these prescription drugs can be a gateway to heroin use and other drug abuses; and so, particularly when it comes to our veterans, we need to make sure that we do whatever possible to prevent this kind of overuse and abuse. I know that alternate care, which we will discuss today, is integral to that effort.

Thank you very much, Mr. Chairman.

Chairman SANDERS. Thank you, Senator Blumenthal.

Senator Isakson.

STATEMENT OF HON. JOHNNY ISAKSON, U.S. SENATOR FROM GEORGIA

Senator ISAKSON. Well, Chairman Sanders, thank you for calling this hearing. I want to echo the words of Ranking Member Burr, yourself, and Senator Blumenthal that the Arizona situation is troubling for all of us.

I am glad we are going to get to the bottom of it. I hope we will do so as expeditiously as possible, and then I hope we can take action to help support VA in finding out where there is a problem, if there is one, and then correcting it.

Dr. Petzel and I have become close friends over the last 8 to 9 months because of incidences that neither one of us wish would have happened. His quick response in Atlanta has been greatly appreciated. His response at the VA hospital in Augusta has been greatly appreciated, and the fact that he is going to be visiting in the next week, I think this weekend, again is very much appreciated and his attention to those matters.

The VA situation we had in Augusta 2 or 3 years ago: the concern about, sterilization of colonoscopy and endoscopy equipment, the difficulty that we had in Atlanta with the suicide situation and the postponement or untimely following of mental health patients; and now what has happened in Arizona should be a warning call for all of us.

I believe we have 340,000 great employees at VA. They do a tremendous job; and as the Chairman and Ranking Member said, I am very proud of what they do. But if there is a growing culture that believes it does not matter or it is not as important or our care is not as important as we think it should be, we need to nip that in the bud and see to it VA is to every veteran and to this country what it was promised to and what it must be.

I think it is important and incumbent upon this Committee to get to the bottom, wherever the facts lead us, and to get the leadership of VA to go with us so that hand-in-hand we can correct the inequities that are going on.

My last point is this. Pharmaceutical therapy is a godsend in terms of pain, in terms of management of disease and other chronic ailments. But it also can interact inappropriately with other drugs for other ailments. It can also be overprescribed. It also can mask a greater problem, particularly with regard to mental health.

This is a terribly important hearing today. I am not a person of medicine nor a person of science but I am familiar enough with what goes on in terms of drug abuse and one drug leading to another, that we cannot allow ourselves to take the easy way out in terms of pain management or therapy for our veterans.

We need to always be looking for the long-term benefit of that veteran, not just the short-term easing of pain when we are prescribing the power opiates that we are talking about today.

Thank you for calling this hearing, Mr. Chairman.

Chairman SANDERS. Senator Isakson, thank you very much for your very apt and important remarks. I agree with virtually everything you said.

What I want to do now, if it is alright with the Committee, is to introduce our panelists, but I did want to give Dr. Petzel a minute or two to address concerns about Arizona. I want the main focus of this hearing to stay on overmedication while there is interest about what is happening in Arizona.

Dr. Petzel, could you briefly give us your understanding of the situation there?

Dr. PETZEL. Thank you very much, Chairman Sanders.

First of all, it is important to state that we do care very deeply about the care of every single veteran that we are privileged to serve. They have earned and they deserve the absolute highest quality care that we can provide.

We take these allegations, as all of you do, very seriously. That is why we have asked the independent office of VA's IG to go there and do an objective, independent, complete review as to exactly what has occurred.

We also sent, from VHA, a team to Phoenix early to review the appointment and scheduling processes, and I need to say that to-date we found no evidence of a secret list and we have found no patients who have died because they have been on a wait list.

We think it is very important that the inspector general be allowed to finish their investigation before we rush to judgment as to what has actually happened in Phoenix.

The other important point is that when an incident like this occurs, as with colonoscopies and mental health consults that were mentioned earlier, we conduct a thorough systemwide look which we are in the process of doing now with scheduling and wait lists, seeing if the alleged practices are not occurring at any one of our other 150 medical centers.

If the allegations are true, they are absolutely unacceptable and we—if the inspector general does confirm and substantiate these claims—we are going to take swift and very appropriate action.

The last point is that the veterans deserve to have full faith in their VA health care system. VA facilities are committed to transparency. We undergo multiple external and independent reviews and every year we are committed to ensuring our veteran community and the public that VA hospitals are safe and that the quality of care there is high.

Finally, as has been mentioned by several of you, we do appreciate the hard work and the dedication of all of our employees. These people are committed to the person to providing, again, the best care possible to these veterans who have earned and who deserve that care.

Thank you.

Chairman SANDERS. OK. Thank you very much, Dr. Petzel.

I thought it was important we deal with that issue briefly. Now, let us focus on the issue at hand which is overmedication problems and solutions. In order to address that issue, we have two excellent panels.

Our first panel will include Dr. Petzel, who is the Under Secretary for Health, Veterans Health Administration, Department of Veterans' Affairs; accompanied by Dr. Tracy Gaudet, who is the Director, Office of Patient Centered Care and Cultural Transformation. Dr. Peter Marshall, Director of Primary Care Pain Management at the Minneapolis VA medical center.

Brigadier General Norvell V. Coots, Deputy Commanding General, U.S. Army Medical Command and Assistant Surgeon General for Force Projection, Office of the Surgeon General; and he is accompanied by Colonel Kevin T. Galloway, Program Director, Army Pain Management Program.

We also have Dr. Josephine Briggs, Director of the National Center for Complementary and Alternative Medicine, National Institutes of Health.

So, thank you all very much for being with us; and Dr. Petzel, you may begin.

STATEMENT OF ROBERT PETZEL, M.D., UNDER SECRETARY FOR HEALTH, VETERANS HEALTH ADMINISTRATION, U.S. DEPARTMENT OF VETERANS AFFAIRS; ACCOMPANIED BY TRACY GAUDET, M.D., DIRECTOR, OFFICE OF PATIENT CENTERED CARE AND CULTURAL TRANSFORMATION AND PETER MARSHALL, M.D., DIRECTOR OF PRIMARY CARE PAIN MANAGEMENT, MINNEAPOLIS VA MEDICAL CENTER

Dr. PETZEL. Good morning, Chairman Sanders, Ranking Member Burr, and the Members of the Committee.

I want to thank you for the opportunity to participate in this hearing to discuss the Department of Veterans Affairs' pain management and opioid safety programs, our use of complementary and alternative medicine, and psychotropic drug safety. I am accompanied today by Dr. Gaudet as was mentioned earlier and by Dr. Peter Marshall.

Before I begin, I want to express my joy at hearing that Senator Boozman is recuperating well. We wish him a speedy recovery and look forward to him participating again in the affairs of this Committee.

Let me begin today by acknowledging all of our Nation's veterans who suffer from chronic and acute pain. The burden of pain on veterans is considerable. Studies say that more that 50 percent of all veterans receiving care at the VA are affected by some type of chronic pain, much of it being musculoskeletal.

Six elements of effective pain control include the safe and effective use of pain care to enhance the quality of life and the satisfaction of veterans that are living with chronic pain.

VA's concept of safe and effective pain care follow these six essential elements. Education of veterans and family members about good pain care. Education of the treatment teams about good pain care. Developing non-pharmacological and self-management approaches. Safe and evidence-based use of all interventions and medications including opioids. Developing effective modalities for bringing pain care, especially expertise, to the veteran when needed. And finally, monitoring pain care efficacy at both the individual veteran level and at the system level.

VA recently developed and implemented an innovative opioid safety program. This program uniquely combines feedback to providers at facilities on their prescribing practices with education and training to ensure opioid pain medications are used safely, effectively, and judiciously across our entire system.

The purpose of the initiative is to help ensure that pain management is addressed thoughtfully, compassionately, and safely. This initiative holds considerable promise for mitigating the risks of harm among veterans receiving long-term opioid therapy, for promoting provider competence and safe prescribing of opioids, and in promoting veteran-centered, evidence-based, coordinated, disciplined, multi-disciplinary pain care for chronic pain.

For cases where veterans have developed problems with opioid abuse and addiction, VA offers effective evidence-based treatments for opioid use disorder. Intensive treatments consisting of options for evidence-based psychotherapy and effective pharmacological therapy for opioid use disorder is available at all of our VA medical centers to help facilitate veterans' recovery.

Recognizing that psycho-pharmacological treatments for mental health conditions require on-going efforts in quality improvement, VA is implementing a psychosocial drug safety initiative.

It addresses pharmacological treatments across the range of mental health conditions including PTSD, depression, schizophrenia, bipolar disorder, substance abuse disorder, and many other mental health conditions.

This psychotropic drug initiative is designed to identify overuse, underuse, and inappropriate use of these drugs by reviewing provider prescribing habits, patient use, and providing feedback to providers about their use of these medications and education about the appropriate use when we do find that the use is inappropriate.

Key leadership has identified as its number 1 strategic goal to provide veteran patients with personalized, proactive, patient-driven health care. This approach to health prioritizes the veteran and their values and partners with them to personalize the strategies to optimize their health, healing, and sense of well-being.

Many of the strategies that may be of benefit extend beyond what we conventionally address or provide by the health care system. Integrative medicine, which includes complementary and alternative medicine, provides a framework that aligns with this goal of personalized, proactive, patient-drive care.

There is a growing evidence for the effectiveness of non-pharmacological approaches as part of a comprehensive plan for chronic pain. These include acupuncture, massage, chiropractic care, mindfulness meditation, exercise therapy, relaxation therapies, and yoga. These are all being increasingly made available to our veteran patients.

Mr. Chairman, we know our work to improve veteran care through accessible, safe, and effective pain management service is an ongoing task and is not yet finished.

However, we are confident that we are developing and implementing programs that are responsive to veteran needs. We appreciate your support in identifying and resolving these challenges as we find new ways to care for America's veterans.

Mr. Chairman, this concludes my testimony. My colleagues and I are prepared to answer your questions.

[The prepared statement of Dr. Petzel follows:]

PREPARED STATEMENT OF DR. ROBERT PETZEL, UNDER SECRETARY FOR HEALTH, VETERANS HEALTH ADMINISTRATION (VHA), U.S. DEPARTMENT OF VETERANS AFFAIRS

Good morning, Chairman Sanders, Ranking Member Burr, and Members of the Committee. Thank you for the opportunity to participate in this hearing and to discuss the Department of Veterans Affairs' (VA) pain management programs and the use of complementary and alternative medicine. I am accompanied today by Dr. Tracy Gaudet, Director of Office of Patient Centered Care & Cultural Transformation, and Dr. Peter Marshall, Director of Primary Care Pain Management.

The challenges related to living with chronic pain and providing safe and effective pain care are by no means unique to Veterans and the VA health care system. As described in the 2011 Institute of Medicine (IOM) report, "Relieving Pain in America: A Blueprint for Transforming Prevention, Care, Education, and Research,"[1] pain is a public health challenge that affects millions of Americans and is increasing in prevalence. Pain contributes to morbidity, mortality, and disability across our Nation and the costs of pain can be measured both in terms of human suffering as well as economic impact. The IOM estimated that chronic pain alone affects 100 million United States citizens and that the cost of pain in the United States is at least $560–$635 billion each year, which is the combined cost of lost productivity and the incremental cost of health care.

CHRONIC PAIN IN VETERANS

The burden of pain on the Veteran population is considerable. We know that Veterans have much higher rates of chronic pain than the general population, with more than 50 percent of all Veterans enrolled and receiving care at VA affected by chronic pain.[2] Chronic pain is the most common medical problem in Veterans returning from the last decade of conflict (almost 60 percent).[3] Many of these Veterans have survived serious and at times catastrophic injuries frequently a result of roadside bombs and other blast injuries. These events can result in multiple physical traumas including amputations and spinal cord injuries as well as concomitant psychological trauma which can compound chronic pain concerns. Often these Veterans require a combination of strategies for the effective management of pain, which may include treatment with opioid analgesics. That makes pain management a very important clinical issue for VA. Further, the treatment of pain is highly complex, and in the recent past, health care providers have often been accused of undertreating the pain that patients suffer. Getting the balance right is a challenge that we continue to work toward.

In 2010, VA and the Department of Defense (DOD) published evidence-based Clinical Practice Guidelines for the use of chronic opioid therapy in chronic pain. The guidelines reserve the use of chronic opioids for patients with moderate to severe pain who have not responded to, or responded only partially to, clinically indicated, evidence-based pain management strategies of lower risk, and who also may benefit from a trial of opioids to improve pain control in the service of improving function and quality of life.

We also know that the long-term use of opioids is associated with significant risks, and can complicate health care for Veterans with Posttraumatic Stress Disorder (PTSD), depression, Traumatic Brain Injury (TBI) and family stress—all common in Veterans returning from the battlefield, and in Veterans with substance use disorders. Chronic pain in Veterans is often accompanied by co-morbid mental health conditions (up to 50 percent in some cohorts) caused by the psychological trauma of war, as well as neurological disorders, such as TBI caused by blast and concussion injuries. In fact, one study documented that more that 40 percent of Veterans admitted to a polytrauma unit in VHA suffered all three conditions together—chronic pain, PTSD, and post-concussive syndrome.[4]

In addition to these newly injured Veterans suffering from chronic pain conditions and neuropsychological conditions, VA cares for millions of Veterans from prior conflicts, who along with chronic pain and psychological conditions resulting from their earlier combat experiences, are now developing health concerns related to aging, such as cancer, neuropathies, spinal disease, and arthritis, all of which may be accompanied by chronic and at times debilitating pain. All of these Veterans deserve safe and effective pain care that may include the use of opioid analgesics when clinically appropriate.

Thus, VA cares for a population that suffers much higher rates of chronic pain than the civilian population, and also experiences much higher rates of co-morbidities (PTSD, depression, TBI) and socioeconomic dynamics (family stress, disability, joblessness) that contribute to the complexity and challenges of pain management with opioids.[5] So even as more Veterans have the kind of severe and dis-

---

[1] Institute of Medicine. 2011. Relieving Pain in America: A Blueprint for Transforming Pain Prevention, Care, Education and Research. Washington, DC: The National Academies Press.
[2] Gironda, R.J., Clark, M.E., Massengale, J.P., & Walker, R.L. (2006).. Pain among Veterans of Operations Enduring Freedom and Iraqi Freedom. Pain Medicine, 7, 339–343.
[3] Veterans Health Administration (2013). Analysis of VA health care utilization among Operation Enduring Freedom (OEF), Operation Iraqi Freedom (OIF), and Operation New Dawn (OND) Veterans. Washington, DC: Department of Veterans Affairs.
[4] Lew, H.L., Otis, J.D., Tun, C., Kerns, R.D., Clark, M.E., & Cifu, D.X. (2009). Prevalence of chronic pain, Post Traumatic Stress Disorder, and post-concussive syndrome in OEF/OIF veterans: The polytrauma clinical triad. *Journal of Rehabilitation Research and Development, 46,* 697–702.
[5] See citations 3 and 4.

abling pain conditions that require stronger treatments such as opioids, so do more of them have increased risk for overdose complicated by depression, PTSD and substance use disorders.

In recognition of the seriousness of the impact of chronic pain on our Veterans' health and quality of life, VHA was among one of the first health systems in the country to establish a robust policy on chronic pain management and to implement a system-wide approach to addressing the risks of opioid analgesia.

I would like to at this time outline our approach to this pain care transformation. I will highlight VA's current pain management strategies as well as actions being taken to improve the management of chronic pain, including the safe use of opioid analgesics, the prevalence and use of opioid therapy to manage chronic pain in high risk Veterans, the challenges of prescription drug diversion [6] and substance use disorders among Veterans, and efforts being made to broaden non-pharmacological approaches to pain care. I will also describe some of the best pain care practices across the VA health care system.

VA'S PAIN CARE MISSION

VA's mission relative to pain care is simple: safe and effective pain care to enhance the quality of life and satisfaction of all Veterans living with chronic pain.

VA's concept of safe and effective pain care includes the following six essential elements:

1. Education of Veterans and family members about good pain care;
2. Education of the treatment teams about good pain care;
3. Developing non-pharmacological and self-management approaches;
4. Safe and evidence-based use of all interventions and medications, including opioids;
5. Developing effective modalities for bringing pain care specialty expertise to the Veteran; and
6. Monitoring pain care efficacy at the individual and system level.

As a blueprint for implementing these principles throughout the system,[7] VHA Pain Management Directive 2009–053 [8] was published in October 2009 to provide uniform guidelines and procedures for providing pain management care. These include standards for pain assessment and treatment, including use of opioid therapy when clinically appropriate, for evaluation of outcomes and quality of pain management, and for clinician competence and expertise in pain management. Since publication of the Pain Management Directive, a dissemination and implementation plan has been enacted that supports the following:

• Comprehensive staffing and training plans for providers and staff;
• Comprehensive patient/family education plans to empower Veterans in pain management;
• Development of new tools and resources to support the pain management strategy; and
• Enhanced efforts to strengthen communication between VA's Central Office (VACO) and leadership from facilities [9] and Veterans Integrated Service Networks (VISN).

Following the guidance of the VHA National Pain Management Strategy, and in compliance with generally accepted pain management standards of care, the Directive provides policy and procedures for the improvement of pain management through implementation of the Stepped Care Model for Pain Management (SCM-PM), the single standard of pain care for VHA, central to ensuring Veterans receive appropriate pain management services. The Directive also requires tracking opioid use and implementing strong practices in risk management to improve Veterans' safety.

To establish the six essential elements of good pain care listed above, numerous modalities have been recently implemented or are in the process of implementation throughout the VHA, including: pain schools, tele-pain schools, apps and web based modules for patient and family education; case based audio conferences, Rural Health Initiative and VeHU trainings, Nation-wide community of practice calls and

---

[6] Diversion is the use of prescription drugs for recreational purposes.

[7] The overall objective of the national strategy is to develop a comprehensive, multicultural, integrated, system-wide approach pain management that reduces pain and suffering and improves quality of life for Veterans experiencing acute and chronic pain associated with a wide range of injuries and illnesses, including terminal illness.

[8] www.va.gov/vhapublications/viewpublication.asp?pub_id=2781

[9] The term "facilities" or "facility" refers to VA's 151 medical centers, hospitals, or health care systems.

numerous other training initiatives to educate and train teams; developing Cognitive Behavioral Therapy (CBT) in primary care, tele-CBT, self-management strategies and complementary and integrative medicine modalities; a number of initiatives to address opioid prescribing which I will discuss shortly; e-consultation, Specialty Care Access Network-Extension for Community Healthcare Outcomes (SCAN-ECHO), and telemedicine to bring pain care expertise to all settings; and pain dashboards to monitor care at the individual and populations levels.

VA facilities are now increasingly leveraging their video conferencing capabilities to reach Veterans in the community based outpatient clinics (CBOC) both rural and highly rural to provide group and individual visits for pain schools, evidence based CBT, smoking cessation, and weight loss through the MOVE program all important for the self-care and self-management skills needed as part of a chronic pain care plan.

A particularly exciting initiative is the development of a pain management application for smart phones that will be used by Veterans and their care partners to develop pain self-management skills. This tool, called VA Pain Coach, will eventually interface with VHA's Electronic Health Record (EHR), with appropriate privacy protections, allowing Veteran-reported information about pain, functioning, and other key elements in a secure mobile application environment to be securely stored and accessible to clinicians. VA Pain Coach, which is part of a suite of VA applications called ''Clinic in Hand,'' has just finished a one-year pilot test phase with 1150 Operation Enduring Freedom/Operation Iraqi Freedom/Operation New Dawn Veterans and their caregivers and is now being converted to HTML 5 and will be available for smart phones, tablets and as a web based application. In the future, a complementary initiative will build a clinician-facing application that will enhance the capacity of clinicians and Veterans to share in monitoring, decisionmaking, treatment planning, and reassessment of pain management interventions.

THE PATIENT ALIGNED CARE TEAM (PACT): THE CORE OF THE STEPPED CARE MODEL

The VA approach to pain care mirrors its approaches to all health care concerns: care is increasingly personalized, proactive and patient driven. Chronic pain, as is the case with all chronic health conditions, is most safely and effectively addressed using a biopsychosocial model in which all aspect of the Veterans health and well-being are included in both the assessment and management of the condition: physical health, psychological health and social health. The basic platform for providing such care is the Veteran's PACT, or patient aligned care team, supported by pain and other specialists. PACT is a partnership between the Veteran and the health care team, which emphasizes prevention, health promotion, and self-management. Veterans are the center of the care team and the PACT teamlet, which includes at its core a primary care provider, nurse care manager, clinical associate, and clerical associate. Core pain teams in PACT often add a behavioral health clinician and pharmacist to help address the complexity of pain management.

THE PAIN MEDICINE SPECIALTY TEAM: SPECIALTY CARE ACCESS SUPPORTING PACT

PACT access to consultation and collaborative care with interdisciplinary pain specialty teams is critical. VHA's Pain Medicine Specialty Team Workgroup, chartered on January 26, 2012, provides standards for pain specialty care services and support of PACT pain management in the Stepped Care Model. Key areas of focus include the development of collaborative care models and participation in provider and team education through telehealth, e-consults, and SCAN-ECHO. VA SCAN-ECHO pain experts provide didactics and case-based learning to PACT members using videoconferencing technologies to strengthen the competencies of providers in pain management. More than 95 percent of VHA facilities have specialty pain clinics with documented yearly increases in use and capacity.

VHA PAIN MANAGEMENT CENTERS: DEVELOPING AND PROMULGATING STRONG PRACTICES

The complexity of managing chronic pain may require a more intensive and structured approach to care than can be provided in the primary care or specialty pain medicine clinics. To address the need for tertiary care pain services, on December 15, 2010, the VHA charted the Interdisciplinary Pain Management Workgroup to assist Veterans Integrated Service Network (VISN) Directors in determining the need for tertiary pain care and pain rehabilitation services. As of January 2014, VA has ten sites in seven VISNs with Commission on Accreditation of Rehabilitation Facilities (CARF)-accredited tertiary care pain rehabilitation programs, an increase from only 2 programs in 2009, with 11 more sites in active preparation or actually applying for CARF status. These Centers have the capacity for providing advanced pain medicine diagnostics, surgical and interventional procedures, and in addition provide intensive, integrated chronic pain rehabilitation for Veterans with complex, co-morbid, or treatment refractory conditions.

VHA is in process of greatly expanding access to such Chronic Pain Rehabilitation Centers. Pursuant to the expectation that every VISN shall have at least one CARF-accredited tertiary, interdisciplinary pain care program no later than September 30, 2014, the long-standing CARF Center at the James Haley Veterans Hospital in Tampa, one of only two multidisciplinary pain management centers that has been twice recognized by the American Pain Society as a Clinical Center of Excellence (the other being a program at Stanford University), has provided direct training to VISN teams from across VHA who wish to start CARF programs. Some VISNs may eventually have 2 or more such programs. In addition, there is an ongoing system-wide education effort, using the expertise at these Centers and in other facilities, to educate physicians in Primary Care PACT and other providers taking care of Veterans with chronic pain conditions about Chronic Pain Rehabilitation approaches.

IMPLEMENTING THE STEPPED CARE MODEL IN VHA

To help manage the implementation of the Stepped Care Model, VHA's National Pain Management Program Office (NPMPO) works closely with other VHA national offices such as pharmacy, mental health, and primary care. Other collaborations include NPMPO's partnership with Women's Health Services to develop a strategic plan to strengthen the capacity for women Veteran pain management services. NPMPO also relies on consultation with the interdisciplinary National Pain Management Strategy Coordinating Committee, consisting of members of all relevant clinical offices/programs in VHA, and meets regularly with all VISN Pain Points of Contact (POC). VISN POCs in turn meet regularly with Facility POCs in their VISN.

The role of the Pain POCs, at the VISN and at the facility level, is primarily to coordinate efforts in regard to pain management from an administrative side. The Pain POCs are expected to work closely with the Pain specialists at each facility within the facility Pain Management Committee. This structure creates a two-way communication of successful 'best practices' in the field, which are then communicated nationally, as well as advice and support on policy implementation. The Pain POCs are not the point of contact for clinical issues regarding individual patients. With regards to evaluation and treatment, a Veteran's clinical point of contact for their individual pain needs is their primary care provider within the PACT. As necessary, the pain medicine specialty team at the facility would work in collaboration.

STEPPED CARE MODEL FOR PAIN MANAGEMENT

As mentioned earlier, SCM-PM is the single standard of pain care for VHA to ensure Veterans receive appropriate pain management services. Specifically, SCM-PM provides for assessment and management of pain conditions in the primary care setting. This is supported by timely access to secondary consultation from pain medicine, behavioral health, physical medicine and rehabilitation, specialty consultation, and care by coordination with palliative care, tertiary care, advanced diagnostic and medical management, and rehabilitation services for complex cases involving co-morbidities such as mental health disorders and TBI.

In FY 2012, VHA made several important investments in implementing the SCM-PM. Major transformational initiatives support the objectives of building capacity for enhanced pain management in the primary care setting, including education of Veterans and caregivers in self-management, as well as promoting equitable and timely access to specialty pain care services.

There are other important efforts contributing to the implementation of SCM-PM in VHA facilities. Current initiatives focus on empowering Veterans in their pain management, and expanding capacity for Veterans to receive evidence-based psychological services as a component of a comprehensive and integrated plan for pain management. For example, during FY 2012, the VHA National Telemental Health Center expanded its capacity to deliver face-to-face, psychological services to Veterans remotely via high-speed videoconferencing links. This initiative not only emphasizes the delivery of cognitive behavior therapy for Veterans with chronic pain, but also promotes pain self-management, leading to reductions in pain and improvements in physical functioning and emotional well-being.

Additionally, a Primary Care and Pain Management Task Force is developing a comprehensive strategic and tactical plan for promoting full implementation of the SCM-PM in the Primary Care setting, and it continues to work on several products in support of this effort. For instance, the Task Force is continuing to expand its network of facility- level Primary Care Pain Management points of contact (Pain Champions) who meet monthly, via teleconference, to identity and share strong practices that have led to improved pain care in primary care settings.

VA's pain management initiatives are designed to optimize timely sharing of new policies and guidance related to pain management standards of care. Of particular importance are VHA's continuing efforts to promote safe and effective use of opioid therapy for pain management, particularly those initiatives designed to mitigate risk for prescription pain medication misuse, abuse, addiction, and diversion.

OPIOID PRESCRIBING

While opioid medications, due to their high risk to benefit ratio in chronic pain, will be playing a less prominent role in chronic pain management in the future, they are a primary focus currently due to the attendant risk of their use, particularly in individuals with some of the co-morbid conditions mentioned above.

To monitor the use of opioids by patients in the VA health care system, VA tracks multi-drug therapy for pain in patients receiving chronic or long-acting opioid therapy for safety and effectiveness. This includes tracking of use of guideline recommended medications for chronic pain (i.e., certain anticonvulsants, tricyclic antidepressants (TCA), and serotonin and norepinephrine reuptake inhibitors (SNRI) which have been shown to be effective for treatment of some chronic pain conditions), and tracking of concurrent prescribing of opioids and certain sedative medications (e.g., benzodiazepines and barbiturates) which can contribute to over sedation and overdose risk when taken with opioids and the other medications for pain listed above.

The prevalence of Veterans using opioids has been measured for Veterans using VHA health care services. For FY 2012, of the 5,779,668 patients seen in VA, 433,136 (7.5 percent) received prescriptions for more than 90 days supply of short-acting opioid medications and 92,297 (1.6 percent) received at least one prescription for a long-acting opioid medication in the year. Thus, since more than 50 percent of Veterans enrolled in VHA suffer from chronic pain, the most common condition in all Veterans, a relatively small percentage of those Veterans are receiving chronic opioid therapy, consistent with the DOD/VA Clinical Practice Guidelines which limit their use to patients with moderate to severe persistent pain that has not responded to other safer alternatives that are clinically appropriate. Of these 525,433 patients that received chronic or long-acting opioid therapy, 79,025 (15 percent) were also prescribed a TCA, 90,066 (17 percent) were also prescribed an SNRI, and 178,361 (34 percent) were also prescribed an anticonvulsant some time in FY 2012.

The co-prescription of either TCAs and SNRIs with opioids is first line therapy for the more severe cases of pain related to nerve damage from disease (e.g., diabetes, cancer) or from injuries (e.g., battlefield blast and projectile injuries with or without limb amputation and spinal cord injury). The numbers above suggest that clinical teams are using medically indicated combinations of medications that are specifically needed for these more severe conditions, which themselves are often co-morbid with musculoskeletal pain such as injuries to joints, spine and muscles. Of note, these prescriptions may or may not have overlapped with the opioid prescription during the year.

Notably, 272,719 (52 percent) of patients on chronic or long-acting opioid therapy received non-medication-based rehabilitative treatments as part of their treatment plan (e.g., physical therapy (32 percent), chiropractic care (1 percent), programs to encourage physical activity (9 percent) or occupational therapy (17 percent), and 241,465 (46 percent) also received behavioral or psychosocial treatment for chronic pain or co-morbid mental health conditions.

These data, showing the use of non-medication treatments, suggest that Veterans are benefiting from VHA's efforts to create access to additional pain treatment modalities besides medication. This is consistent with VA's commitment to transform pain care to a biopsychosocial model [10] that addresses all the factors that by research are demonstrated to affect Veterans' success in chronic pain treatment. Pursuant to this aim, a multimodality, team-based, stepped care model, per VHA Directive 2009–053, is being implemented widely throughout VHA, and in coordination with DOD.

Opioid analgesics may help many patients manage their severe pain when other medications and modalities are ineffective or are only partially effective. However,

---

[10] The Biopsychosocial Model takes the position that the causes and outcomes of many illnesses often involve the interaction of physical and pathophysiologic factors, psychological traits and states, and social-environmental factors. Effective treatment planning accounts for the salience of these factors in the precipitation and perpetuation of illness and illness-related disability.

there may be risks to both individual patients as well as to the surrounding community when these agents are not prescribed or used appropriately. VA has embarked on a two-pronged approach to addressing the challenge of prescription drug diversion and substance use disorders among Veteran patients. One approach is to improve the education and training in pain management and safe opioid prescribing for clinicians and the interdisciplinary teams that provide pain management care for Veterans. A complementary approach involves improving risk management through two systems initiatives.

OPIOID SAFETY INITIATIVE

VA recently developed and implemented an Opioid Safety Initiative (OSI) program to ensure opioid pain medications are used safely, effectively and judiciously. The Opioid Safety Initiative Requirements were issued to the VISN's on April 2, 2014. The purpose of the initiative is to ensure pain management is addressed thoughtfully, compassionately and safely. The nine goals are summarized below:

• Goal One: Educate prescribers of opioid medication regarding effective use of urine drug screening
  • Goal Two: Increase the use of urine drug screening
  • Goal Three: Facilitate use of state prescription databases
  • Goal Four: Establish safe and effective tapering programs for the combination of benzodiazepines and opioids
  • Goal Five: Develop tools to identify higher risk patients
  • Goal Six: Improve prescribing practices around long-acting opioid formulations
  • Goal Seven: Review treatment plans for patients on high doses of opioids
  • Goal Eight: Offer Complementary and Alternative Medicine (CAM) modalities for chronic pain at all facilities
  • Goal Nine: Develop new models of mental health and primary care collaboration to manage opioid and benzodiazepine prescribing in patients with chronic pain

To do this, the initiative leverages the VHA's Electronic Health Record, making visible the totality of opioid use at all levels, patient, provider and facility, in order to identify high-risk situations. The OSI includes key clinical indicators such as the number of unique pharmacy patients dispensed an opioid, unique patients on long-term opioids who receive a urine drug screen, the number of patients receiving an opioid and a benzodiazepine (which puts them at a higher risk of adverse events) and the average dosage per day of opioids such as hydromorphone, methadone, morphine, oxycodone, and oxymorphone. Patients at risk for adverse events from use of opioids are identified through the use of administrative and clinical databases using pre-determined parameters based on published evidence and expert opinion. Providers whose prescribing practices are not aligned with medical evidence/strong practices are provided with counseling, education and support for to improve their care of Veterans with pain. Several aspects to measure the implementation of the Opioid Safety Initiative upon opioid use were underway at the time of the October 10, 2013 hearing and suggested positive impacts:

• Despite an increase in the number of Veterans who were dispensed any medication from a VA pharmacy, (i.e., all pharmacy users) in October 2012 compared to November 2013, 39,088 fewer Veterans received an opioid prescription from VA during that time period.
• Performing urine drug screens is a useful tool to assist in the clinical management of patients receiving long-term opioid therapy. As of November 2013, urine drug screens were performed on 80,294 more patients than in October 2012.
• Whenever clinically feasible, the concomitant use of opioid and benzodiazepine medications should be avoided. In November 2013, 9,609 fewer patients were receiving these drugs at the same time than in October 2012.
• Last, the average dose of selected opioids has begun to decline slightly in VA, demonstrating that prescribing and consumption behaviors are changing.

While these changes may appear to be modest given the size of the VA patient population, they signal an important trend in VA's use of opioids. VA expects this trend to continue as it renews its efforts to promote safe and effective pharmacologic and non-pharmacologic pain management therapies. Very effective programs yielding significant results have been identified (e.g. Minneapolis, Tampa, Columbus), and are being studied as strong practice leaders.

The second system-wide risk management approach to support the Veterans' and public's safety is promulgation of new regulations that enable VHA to participate in state Prescription Drug Monitoring Programs (PDMPs). VA providers can now access the state PDMP for information on prescribing and dispensing of controlled substances to Veterans outside the VA health care system. Participation in PDMPs will enable providers to identify patients who have received non-VA prescriptions for controlled substances, which in turn offers greater opportunity to discuss the effectiveness of these non-VA prescriptions in treating their pain or symptoms. More importantly, information that can be gathered through these programs will help both VA and non-VA providers to prevent harm to patients that could occur if the provider was unaware that a controlled substance medication had been prescribed elsewhere already.

LEVERAGING STRONG PRACTICES TO CHANGE OPIOID PRESCRIBING:
THE MINNEAPOLIS VA MEDICAL CENTER (VAMC)

In summary, there is growing evidence of the successful implementation of a Stepped Care Model for Pain Management in VHA. Importantly, Veterans receiving long term opioid therapy for management of chronic pain are increasingly likely to be receiving this therapy in the context of multidisciplinary and multimodal care that often incorporates physical and occupational therapy and mental health services. All VISNs provide specialty pain clinic services, and the number of Veterans who receive these services has grown steadily for the past five years. Ten facilities now provide CARF accredited pain rehabilitation services, a rapid increase in the availability of these higher specialized pain rehabilitation services for our most complex Veterans with debilitating chronic pain and comorbid mental health disorders.

VA learns from VISNs and VAMCs that are early adopters of implementing evidence-based guidelines and best practices. The Minneapolis VAMC has had great success with decreasing over utilization of opioid pain medications and developing a full range of pain management services. These efforts began with the Minneapolis VA Opioid Safety Initiative in 2011. Strong medical center leadership support led to the development of systems to identify patients on high risk opioids and provide team-based support from pharmacy, primary care, and mental health to develop individualized care plans to decrease high risk opioid use and improve patient safety. Implementing this best practices approach, Minneapolis has seen a nearly 70 percent decrease in high-dose opioid prescribing for chronic non-cancer pain patients. This early success lead to a coordinated effort between Minneapolis VAMC and VISN 23 to expand support for PACT team-based pain management, Step 2 pain consultation services, and rehabilitation focused multidisciplinary pain specialty services. The Minneapolis pain specialty services are now developing state-of-the-art, evidence-based interdisciplinary pain management programs and services, and also providing leadership, guidance, and support for primary care pain management throughout VISN 23 and VHA.

VA is working aggressively to promote the safe and effective use of long-term opioid therapy for Veterans with chronic pain for whom this important therapy is indicated. VA's Opioid Safety Initiative holds considerable promise for mitigating risk for harms among Veterans receiving this therapy, for promoting provider competence in safe prescribing of opioids, and in promoting Veteran-centered, evidence-based, and coordinated multidisciplinary pain care for Veterans with chronic pain. VA's Opioid Safety Initiative Tool provides monthly reports to all VISNs and facilities as to overall opioid prescribing an average dose per day of opioid therapy, which informs facilities of Veterans who are at risk for adverse outcomes and enables remedial steps to reduce those risks as described earlier by the Minneapolis VAMC. Interventions include VISN level, facility level and committees that provide support and education to improve the appropriate opioid risk mitigation for individual providers and facilities. Early evidence of success in reducing overall opioid prescribing and average dose per day of opioid therapy is encouraging.

COMPLEMENTARY AND INTEGRATIVE MEDICINE

VHA leadership has identified as its number one strategic goal "to provide Veterans personalized, proactive, patient-driven health care." Integrative Health (IH), which includes CAM approaches, provides a framework that aligns with personalized, proactive, patient-driven care. There is growing evidence for effectiveness of non-pharmacological approaches as part of a comprehensive care plan for chronic pain which includes acupuncture, massage, yoga and spinal manipulation. These are all being increasingly made available to Veterans.

In 2011, VA's Healthcare Analysis and Information Group published a report on Complementary and Alternative Medicine in VA. At that time, 89 percent of VHA facilities offered some form of CAM/IH; however, there was extensive variability regarding the degree, level, and spectrum of services being offered in VHA. The top reasons for offering CAM/IH included the following:

• Promotion of wellness;
• Patient preferences; and

• Adjunct to chronic disease management.

The most commonly offered CAM/IH modalities in VHA facilities were: Meditation, Stress Management/Relaxation Therapy, Progressive Muscle Relaxation, Biofeedback, and Guided Imagery. The conditions most commonly treated with CAM/IH include: Stress management, Anxiety Disorders, PTSD, Depression, and Back Pain.

In VA, chiropractic care is part of the standard medical benefits and is administratively aligned under Rehabilitation and Prosthetic Services. The number of Veterans receiving chiropractic services in VA has expanded form under 4,000 in FY 2004, to over 26,000 in FY 2013. In addition to clinical services, Rehabilitation and Prosthetic Services is working to develop innovative approaches to foster chiropractic inter-professional education strategies and research projects.

VA recognizes the importance and benefits of recreational therapy in the rehabilitation of Veterans with disabilities. Currently, over 30 VA medical centers across the country participate in therapeutic riding programs. These programs use equine assisted therapeutic activities to promote healing and rehabilitation of Veterans with a variety of disabilities and medical conditions (e.g. Traumatic Brain Injury, polytrauma). VA facilities participating in such programs utilize their locally appropriated funds to support their participation. Facilities can also request supplemental support through the VA Secretary's General Post Fund, a trust fund administered by the Department to support a variety of recreational and religious projects and national rehabilitation special events.

A monthly Integrative Health (IH) community of practice conference call provides VHA facilities national updates, strong practices, and new developments in the field and research findings related to IH.

A key development is a Joint Incentive Fund DOD/VA project to improve Veterans' and Servicemembers' access to CAM, the "Tiered Acupuncture Training Across Clinical Settings" (ATACS) project. ATACS represents VHA's initiative to make evidence-based complementary and alternative medicine therapies widely available to our Veterans throughout VHA. A VHA and DOD network of medical acupuncturists are being identified and trained in Battlefield (auricular) Acupuncture by regional training conferences organized jointly by VHA and DOD. The goal of the project is for them to return to their facilities and VISNs with the skills to train local providers in Battlefield Acupuncture, which has been used successfully in DOD front-line clinics around the world. This initiative ultimately aims to provide all Veterans with access to this intervention, and a wider array of pain management choices generally, when they present with chronic pain.

INTEGRATIVE HEALTH—THE WAY FORWARD

In late 2012, the Under Secretary for Health appointed a Team to review the organizational structure to support implementation of integrative health strategies in VHA. The Team recommended the expansion of the VHA Office of Patient Centered Care and Cultural Transformation's (OPCC&CT) capacity to develop and implement integrative health strategies in clinical activities, education, and research. OPCC&CT is now serving as the lead office in this work, expanding on existing efforts and with active partnerships across the organization. An Acting Director of VHA's Integrative Health Coordinating Center (IHCC) has been named and recruitment for core staff is in process. Additional staffing is being vetted now and that will continue until the program is fully developed.

OPCC&CT has deployed a number of clinical, research, and education strategies to begin developing a more coordinated approach. This includes clinical pilots, work within the existing Centers of Innovations, and close alignment with the Office of Research and Development, as well as creating curricula and expanding education in these areas. VA's Evidence Synthesis program, in conjunction with OPCC&CT and Patient Care Services, is examining the scientific literature on various CAM modalities and presenting the findings in the form of an evidence map. At the present time, reviews are being done on Yoga, Tai Chi, and mindfulness meditation and a review was recently completed on acupuncture. The evidence map on acupuncture showed a positive effect of acupuncture on headaches, migraines, and chronic pain as well as a potential positive effect in multiple domains including depression and insomnia. The information from these reviews will help guide decision on how to best use CAM modalities within VA.

The Whole Health Clinical Education Program, which includes an integrative health focus, launched last year, has received outstanding evaluation feedback from the clinicians and leadership who have taken the course. An online curriculum is under development and will have greater than 40 modules. These have been co-created with VA and the University of Wisconsin, leaders in the field of Integrative Medicine.

Finally, the DOD/VA Health Executive Council (HEC) Pain Management Work Group (PMWG) was chartered to develop a model system of integrated, timely, continuous, and expert pain management for Servicemembers and Veterans. The Work Group participates in VA/DOD Joint Strategic Planning (JSP) process to develop and implement the strategies and performance measures, as outlined in the JSP guidance, and shares responsibility in fostering increased communication regarding functional area between Departments. The Group also identifies and assesses further opportunities for the coordination and sharing of health related services and resource between the Departments. A key development is the HEC PMWG's sponsoring of two Joint Incentive Fund projects to improve Veterans' and Service-members' access to competent pain care in the SCM-PM: the Joint Pain and Education Project (JPEP), and the "Tiered Acupuncture Training Across Clinical Settings" (ATACS) projects.

OVERSIGHT AND ACCOUNTABILITY

Several key responsibilities are articulated in the Pain Management Directive. The Directive establishes a National Pain Management Program Office (NPMPO) in VACO that has the responsibility for policy development, coordination, oversight, and monitoring of VHA's National Pain Strategy. The Directive further authorizes the establishment of a multidisciplinary VHA National Pain Management Strategy Coordinating Committee that supports the Program Office in achieving its strategic goals and objectives. The Committee is comprised of 15 members to include: anesthesiology, employee education, geriatrics and extended care, mental health, neurology, nursing, pain management, patient education, pharmacy benefits management, primary care/internal medicine, quality performance, rehabilitation medicine, research, and women Veterans' health.

The Directive requires VISN Directors to ensure that all facilities establish and implement current pain management policies consistent with this Directive. The NPMPO maintains records of VISN and facility compliance, along with other key organizational requirements contained in the Directive. All VISNs and facilities have appointed National Pain Office pain management points of contact, established multidisciplinary committees, and implemented pain management policies as required by the Directive. Health Care Provider Education and Training

First, as recognized by the IOM in its extensive 2011 review, "Pain in America" and the American Medical Association in its 2010 Report on Pain Medicine[11], and as articulated in VHA's Pain Management Directive in 2009–053, a formal commitment to pain management education and training for all appropriate clinical staff is required.

The Joint Pain and Education Project, JPEP, mentioned earlier, has proposed training faculty in all VA training sites to pursue the implementation of such a curriculum; new generations of providers and other clinicians will themselves ultimately become the practitioners and teachers of good pain care. JPEP will target all levels of learner: the Veteran and his/her family and caregiver; the public; clinicians from all disciplines; specific providers and clinicians in practicing at each level of the SCM-PM: primary care, pain medicine specialty care, and other specialty care. VA is providing national leadership in developing interdisciplinary and discipline-specific competencies for pain management, in developing a system-wide approach to trainings, and in providing leadership roles in national projects to improve pain education and training.

CONCLUSION

Mr. Chairman, I would be the last person to say that we are now right where we want to be with our pain care in VA, but I will be the first person to say that we are well along in the process of getting there. I am confident that we will be setting standards for pain care nationally in the coming years. We are confident that we are building more accessible, safe and effective pain care that will be responsive to the needs of our Veterans and will better serve to enhance the quality of their lives. VA is committed to providing the high quality of care that our Veterans have earned and deserve, and we appreciate the opportunity to appear before you today. My colleagues and I are prepared to respond to any questions you may have.

---

[11] Lippe P.M., Brock C., David J.J., Crossno R., Gitlow S. The First National Pain Medicine Summit—Final Summary Report. Pain Med 2010;11(10):1447–68.

RESPONSE TO POSTHEARING QUESTIONS SUBMITTED BY HON. BERNARD SANDERS TO ROBERT A. PETZEL, MD, UNDER SECRETARY FOR HEALTH, VETERANS HEALTH ADMINISTRATION (VHA), U.S. DEPARTMENT OF VETERANS AFFAIRS

OPIOID SAFETY INITIATIVE

Question 1. How does VA plan to implement the Opioid Safety Initiative system-wide?

Response. The Veterans Health Administration (VHA) has been vigorously pursuing implementation the Opioid Safety Initiative (OSI) to ensure optimal pain management and to safeguard Veterans from harm inherent in high-risk medications such as opioids and benzodiazepines. The objective of OSI is to make the totality of opioid use visible at all levels in the organization with a particular emphasis on identifying and remediating prescribing practices that place Veterans at increased risk for adverse outcomes. To this end, VHA has embarked on a system-wide program of education and training in pain management, opioid safety, access to alternative medical and non-medical treatments for pain, and patient education in self-management. These programs are manifestations of the core principles and policies outlined in the 2009 Directive and are emphasized in the new draft Directive which is in development. In the meantime, Directive 2009–053 remains as VHA policy until replaced with the new Directive. To assist Veterans, providers and clinical teams in achieving OSI goals for safer opioid prescribing practices, an interdisciplinary VHA Task Force assembled a 15 module, peer-reviewed OSI Toolkit that is continually updated as new information becomes available, including new evidence-based practices. The OSI Toolkit is accessible to all VHA clinicians and disseminated widely and repeatedly through multiple communication channels and educational formats to facilitate safe opioid prescribing practices.

a. What is the timeline for full implementation?

Response. While The Opioid Safety Initiative (OSI) was launched in October 2013, it is an on-going endeavor, comprised of multiple inter-disciplinary approaches, which will be constantly evaluated, modified and/or introduced to effective pain management and decrease the risks for complications due to both over- and under-treatment with opioids and other therapies. As an example, VHA OSI Task Force assembled a 15 module, peer-reviewed OSI Toolkit that is continually updated as new information becomes available, including new evidence-based practices.

Question 2. What are the implications of the Opioid Safety Initiative beyond pain care, such as reducing the reliance of medications to treat mental health conditions?

Response. VHA original response: The Opioid Safety Initiative addresses the risks of opioid analgesia comprehensively through a system-wide program with the following aims that include management of Veterans with co-morbid pain and mental health conditions:

• To reduce risks, such as high opioid doses, co-prescribing of benzodiazepines, close monitoring of Veterans with urine drug screens and Veterans with risks such as substance use disorders (addiction) and PTSD.

• To encourage the use of psychological, physical and complementary and alternative medicine (CAM) therapies such as acupuncture and yoga in pain management.

• To provide feedback and educational support for our clinical teams caring for patients with co-morbid pain and mental health disorders.

Question 3. How does VA plan to publicize this initiative—particularly to veterans who may have avoided seeking treatment in the past because of concerns regarding medication?

Response. VHA has embarked on a system-wide program of education and training in pain management, opioid safety, access to alternative medical and non-medical treatments for pain, and patient education in self-management. These programs are manifestations of the core principles and policies outlined in the 2009 Directive and are emphasized in the new draft Directive which is currently in concurrence. In the meantime, Directive 2009–053 remains VHA policy until replaced with the new Directive.

Question 4. One of the goals of the Opioid Safety Initiative is to facilitate use of state prescription databases. In which state prescription databases is VA able to participate? Is VA currently participating in all of the databases where it is able?

Response. As of the date of this response, Prescription Drug Monitoring Program (PDMP) deployment is completed in 29 states, and is scheduled for completion in 6 more states by the end of August 2015. Please note that in 2 of these 6 states—Florida and Oregon—PDMP deployment is very near completion. In Florida, 4 of 6 sites are transmitting and in Oregon, 2 of 3 sites are transmitting. Deployment will occur in 13 other states by December 2016. The longer implementation period for these 13 states is due to their individually customized PDMP requirements that VA is working to satisfy. One state—New Mexico—has advised the Department that it needs to purchase and install new software to support a PDMP, and that its timeline to accomplish this purchase is not yet determined. This issue affects all dispensing pharmacies within New Mexico. VA stands ready to activate the transmission of prescription drug data to New Mexico's PDMP system as soon as the state is ready. Missouri is the only state that has not enacted a PDMP law. The District of Columbia is currently developing its recently enacted PDMP. A complementary effort to PDMP deployment is the issuance of the VHA Directive, Querying State Prescription Drug Monitoring Programs, which we are planning to publish in the coming months. This Directive would establish policy requiring VHA health care provider participation in state PDMPs, consistent with applicable state laws. The Directive would assign responsibility to each facility Director to ensure that local policy and processes are established to support the Directive. Specifically, the Directive would outline when a query is needed, the frequency of a query, and any exclusions. Specifically, the draft would exclude any controlled substance prescription that is a 5 day supply or less without refills and any patient who is enrolled in Hospice care, unless required by state law.

COMPLEMENTARY AND ALTERNATIVE MEDICINE (CAM)

Question 5. VA offers a number of CAM therapies, but they are not necessarily evenly distributed across the system and veterans are not always aware of what's available to them. What is VA doing to more evenly distribute access across the system? What is VA doing to inform veterans their options for CAM therapies? What is VA doing to encourage providers to offer these therapies and how is this being tracked?

Response. VA is committed to offering Veterans more personalized, proactive and patient driven care. This entails better understanding of the needs and desires of Veterans and addressing their health care goals in a more holistic fashion. VHA has established an Integrative Health Coordinating Center whose mission is to help evaluate and where appropriate help integrate Complementary and Integrative Health (CIH) services into VA. In addition, the Office of Patient Centered Care and Cultural Transformation (OPCC&CT) has developed education on Whole Health, which is being disseminated throughout VA. These courses educate providers on how to approach healthcare in a more holistic fashion and educates them on CIH practices and how these may be able to play a part in Veterans healthcare. This education on CIH practices will expand the resources available to providers when they engage their patients in identifying their healthcare goals and the strategies they wish to embark on to attain these goals. As VA offers personalized, proactive, patient-driven care it is through educating providers that we work to ensure that Veterans have a discussion with their provider and discuss the best treatment option including all appropriate therapies including indicated CAM/CIH which is unique to the Veteran and their circumstance. VHA's educational programs for clinical staff are being disseminated in the field. These clinical courses educate providers on how to approach health care in a more holistic way and educates them on CAM therapies available. Other efforts are underway to provide information to Veterans. One example is that OPCC&CT developed an internet site as the focal point for messaging, resource delivery, and community engagement for the patient centered care body of work and the Veteran-facing products developed to educate and communicate with Veterans. Through the Health for Life site, we are providing products that enable Veterans to achieve their greatest health and well-being. OPCC&CT has also trained field implementation teams that are being deployed around the country to work with local leadership to create a culture that supports a whole health, patient-centered model inclusive of CIH services. They have developed an education campaign that includes both internal and external customer facing modules describing the new models of care and services that focus on putting the patient at the center of their care to create a personalized, proactive, patient-driven model.

Question 6. What factors limit VA from further broadening CAM therapies across the VA Health Care System?

Response. The medical benefits package states that VA may offer those services that are in accord with generally accepted standards of medical practice. There are a vast number of Complementary and Integrative Health (CIH) practices, but the evidence base for many of them is limited. Questions remain about the efficacy of many of these practices, who responds to them, how they should be used, and for how long. Although no CIH practice is the gold standard for care, several practices show promise as adjuncts to care. In addition, many CIH practices lack standardized education, training, certification and licensure standards. These factors, combined with a lack of occupational classes for CIH practitioners within VA, pose significant barriers to the hiring of such providers within VA.

DOD/VA COLLABORATION

Question 7. What benefits has VA seen from the standardization of the prescription medication between VA and DOD available to both servicemembers and veterans? Are servicemembers able to continue their existing course of treatment as they transition to VA health care?

Response. Yes, Servicemembers are able to continue their existing course of treatment as they transition to VA health care, unless a change would be warranted based on a VA provider's clinical assessment (i.e., drug is no longer effective, patient's changing medical condition warrants a change, drug is no longer safe given clinical circumstances, etc.). There have been widespread anecdotal reports of Servicemembers' mental health and pain medications being switched due to differences between the VA and DOD drug formularies. However, these anecdotes were not substantiated in a medication continuity pilot evaluation of over 2,000 Servicemembers recently conducted by VA. In this pilot evaluation, VA found that 99% of patients receiving a mental health or pain medication were able to continue those medications despite differences between the VA and DOD formularies. The data from VA's pilot evaluation validates VA's long standing practice of continuing medication therapy started by Department of Defense prescribers. See (http://www.pbm.va.gov/PBM/vacenterformedicationsafety/othervasafetyprojects/DOD—VA—Medication—Continuation—Report.pdf).

Question 8. What other efforts have DOD and VA taken to collaborate and standardize treatment options for servicemembers and veterans for the treatment of chronic pain and mental health conditions?

Response. The DOD/VA Health Executive Council's Pain Management Work Group (HEC PMWG), which meets monthly, was chartered in 2010 to ''actively collaborate in supporting the development of a model system of integrated, timely, continuous, and expert pain management for Servicemembers and Veterans.'' The HEC PMWG has articulated 6 objectives for its present work:

Objective 1—Standardize Pain Measurement. The PMWG has sponsored the development of the Defense and Veterans Pain Rating Scale to improve the measurement of pain. The tool has been validated and published, is in use in multiple military facilities and in civilian hospitals. Additional validation studies continue in DOD and VHA.

Objective 2—Develop a clinical pain support tool and pain data registry. The PASTOR tool, incorporating the NIH ''PROMIS'' patient report outcome measures and computer adaptive testing, is under development and is being piloted in a collaboration between Madigan Army Hospital, NIH, and the University of Washington.

Objective 3—Standardize Suboxone (buprenorphine and naloxone) Prescribing Practices. A common guidance document is developed and VHA and DOD working implementation in each organization.

Objective 4—Develop Medical Drug Testing guidance. The PMWG developed DOD/VHA core guidance and have developed and share clinical education and training in JPEP modules and in the Opioid Safety Initiative Toolkit.

Objective 5—Develop Acupuncture Credentialing guidance. The PMWG developed shared DOD/VHA core guidance for VHA and DOD clinicians and is working implementation of core guidance within their respective organizations

Objective 6—Develop Informed Consent for Long-term Opioid Therapy. The VHA developed and approved a patient education document, ''Taking Opioids Responsibly,'' to assist in the informed consent process, and the DOD is evaluating the VHA document for implementation in DOD.

Currently there are two Joint Investment Fund (JIF) supported projects to improve the competencies of our workforce across both systems:

• The Joint Pain Education and Training Project (JPEP).
  – Has developed 35 optional evidence-based training modules in pain management for use in its multiple pain education programs to help standardize pain management education and training across the two health systems and to support and educate clinicians and Veterans about safe and effective stepped pain management, including use of opioids.
  – JPEP modules are being used for primary care residency training and for practicing clinicians and clinical teams being trained by the Pain Mini-resi-

dency, Pain SCAN ECHO, asynchronous web-based courses, and Community of Practice conferences.

— All these programs reach across the VHA to train primary care providers in all settings in the assessment and treatment of pain and in the use of patient education in self-management, the use of multiple modalities such as behavioral, integrative medicine, and physical therapies and the use of consultant specialists in pain, mental health, and CAM.

— On the topic of opioids safety, for example, these programs have presentations on universal precautions and risk management, including clinical evaluation, written informed consent, screening such as urine drug monitoring, use of state prescription monitoring programs, and safe tapering.

• The Tiered Acupuncture Training Across Clinical Settings (ATACS)

— Has trained more than 1290 front-line providers in the VA and DOD in Battlefield Acupuncture as well as dozens of physicians in medical acupuncture.

— Represents VHA's initiative to make evidence-based complementary and alternative medical therapies widely available to our Veterans throughout VHA.

— Provides Veterans with a wider array of pain management choices when they present with chronic pain.

ACUPUNCTURE TRAINING

Question 9. How would the Joint Incentive Fund Project to implement a standardized acupuncture training and sustainment model across DOD and VA medical facilities improve acupuncture services VA provides veterans? When can we expect system-wide implementation of this joint model?

Response. By providing standardized training in the short course for Battlefield (auricular) Acupuncture (BFA) to hundreds of providers across the system, and by credentialing trainees to add BA to their pain management toolbox, these providers will be able to use this treatment as one of many they have to offer Veterans with pain. The physicians being trained in Medical Acupuncture will also be trained as BFA Faculty, so they can train their local facility providers in BFA to sustain the program's development system-wide.

Question 10. How many providers are trained in acupuncture already working in the VA Health Care System? How many of these providers are exclusively providing acupuncture? What is the average number of hours each provider trained in acupuncture offers this therapy each week?

Response. We do not have information on the number of providers based at facilities who provide acupuncture or how many hours a week therapy is provided. However, from the 2015 Healthcare analysis and information group survey on VA Complementary and Integrative Health practices, we do know that 79 facilities offer acupuncture services primarily performed by physician-trained acupuncturists as a part of their duties at least a half day per week up to several times a week.

Question 11. What efforts are being made to ensure an adequate number are available to treat veterans once the joint model is implemented?

Response. At the current time, physicians and chiropractors are the only VHA occupations with scopes of practice that include acupuncture. As a result, the availability of trained acupuncture providers within VA is limited. VA continues to support the training of physicians in acupuncture, but is also pursuing the development of a licensed acupuncturist occupational class within VHA. The addition of licensed acupuncturists to VHA occupations will expand VHA's ability to hire trained acupuncture providers.

PAIN MANAGEMENT DIRECTIVE

Question 12. On October 28, 2009, VA issued the Pain Management Directive to improve VHA's processes for treating and managing chronic pain. How has system-wide implementation of the National Pain Management Strategy—as required by the Pain Management Directive—improved VA's approach to pain management?

Response. The implementation of Stepped Care has increased resources for primary care pain management, such as behavioral health clinicians, access to CAM, access to multidisciplinary pain specialty clinics, and access to tertiary care Commission on Accreditation of Rehabilitation Facilities (CARF) rehabilitation programs.

Question 13. Does VA plan to extend the Pain Management Directive? If not, please explain why not. If so, please explain whether it will be extended in its current form or if changes will be made.

Response. Yes, a new Directive has been drafted and is undergoing VHA Concurrence. Until which time the new Directive is approved, the current Pain Management Directive will remain in effect.

————

RESPONSE TO POSTHEARING QUESTIONS SUBMITTED BY HON. MARK BEGICH TO ROBERT A. PETZEL, MD, UNDER SECRETARY FOR HEALTH, VETERANS HEALTH ADMINISTRATION (VHA), U.S. DEPARTMENT OF VETERANS AFFAIRS

Question 14. My office has received casework from veterans who have severe PTSD issues that affect their day to day life, and say I quote "I'm pretty much done with medications." They have asked for Hero Dogs, who raise and train service dogs and places them free of charge with our Nation's Veterans to improve quality of life and restore independence. Veterans with disabilities have given enough.

Tell me what the VA is doing with expanding service/therapy dogs; I think this would be a cheaper option and a safer option rather than treating with opioids and other drugs.

Response. Veteran preference is an important consideration when choosing a therapeutic approach to treat PTSD. Effective cognitive behavioral therapies are made available to every Veteran who seeks VA care for PTSD. VA is currently attempting to find ways to increase Veteran engagement with these treatment modalities and increase the likelihood that Veterans remain in treatment until remission or significant clinical improvement is accomplished. While dogs and other animals can provide great comfort and companionship, and we do not disagree with Veterans' subjective accounts that service dogs have improved the quality of their lives. At this time, there is not sufficient evidence that animals are effective in the treatment of mental health conditions, including Post Traumatic Stress Disorder (PTSD). Consequently, VA does not provide service dog benefits for mental health service dogs. VA is currently evaluating the efficacy of mental health service dogs pursuant to a congressionally mandated study to learn whether service dogs and/or emotional support dogs can be effective in treating or rehabilitating persons with PTSD. The study, expected to take several years to complete, is currently ongoing at three sites (Atlanta, GA; Iowa City, IA; and Portland, OR) and has begun pairing enrolled Veterans with dogs.

Question 15. The following is from a veteran in Kenai: "I'm on ten different types of medications that deal with sleep, back pain, depression, anxiety, blood pressure, and inflammation * * *. I've really lost count of what I'm taking. I'm sick of it. I don't want to take any more medications. I would like to see if we can make a push for the VA to fund holistic style medical treatments. I believe in these, and I believe that they are cheaper rather than pushing big pharma on us. I for one am sick of it and would rather live in a state of depression and anxiety as opposed to taking 10+ pills a day. I'm also battling with the VA for an increase in VET benefits. They have turned down request for shoulder pain connected disability; they've turned down requests for increase in ringing in my ears but will give me pills!"

I am glad the VA and the Committee is addressing this, it is very real, and how would you respond to this veteran?

Response. Thank you for raising this important point. The problems you mention affect our entire nation and this is an issue we are challenged to manage effectively for our Veterans as well. The VA is actively addressing these problems in multiple ways, as well as contributing to the national effort, outlined in the National Pain Strategy, to improve the education and training of all health professionals, including those who eventually will care for our Veterans and military. The potential for side effects and toxicity increases when medications that affect the central nervous system (the brain and spinal cord) are prescribed together for symptoms of different, but sometimes related, conditions such as sleep disorders, chronic pain conditions, anxiety and depression disorders, Traumatic Brain Injury (TBI) and PTSD. To help combat this problem the VA can take advantage of its unique combination of assets, such as its electronic medical record and its Veterans Health Administration (VHA)-wide communication and education systems which reach all facilities and providers.

VHA has developed a new tool, the Opioid Therapy Risk Report (OTTR), which is available now to all VHA Primary Care clinicians when treating a Veteran with opioid therapy for chronic pain. This report provides information about the dosages of opioid analgesics and other centrally active medications such as benzodiazepines, significant medical and psychiatric problems that could contribute to an adverse drug reaction, and monitoring data to aid in the review and management of complex patients. OTTR is right on the dashboard of the electronic medical record, which enables VA providers to review this pertinent clinical data related to pain treatment all in one place while actually talking to patients about their symptoms and medications. As a result, Veterans are afforded a comprehensive Veteran-centered and more efficient level of pain management not previously available to Primary Care providers. VHA is actively deploying training aids to providers and facilities to familiarize them with how to utilize this tool in their daily practice.

VHA has formalized several education and academic detailing projects that provide all VA prescribers and facilities guidance and education on safe symptom management. One program is the OSI, which monitors reductions in potential risks such as prescribing opioids and benzodiazepines together or high doses of opioids, monitors how facilities are increasing the use of evidence-based alternative treatments such as cognitive behavioral therapies and integrative medicine (CAM) (which are now required to be available in all facilities as alternatives to medication), and also provides feedback and support for providers whose prescribing profiles do not meet acceptable clinical standards. An OSI Toolkit with detailed education and guidance for both providers and patients is available on the VA's Pain Management Intranet and Internet sites and has been widely presented throughout the VHA in multiple educational formats and communications. For example, the Toolkit has detailed instructions about guiding safe medication tapers when clinically indicated.

Programs such as the ATACS are presently training physicians in medical acupuncture and providers in "battlefield (auricular) acupuncture" across both systems. Already 1,293 Providers have been trained in battlefield acupuncture in military treatment facilities VA hospitals across the country.

————

RESPONSE TO POSTHEARING QUESTIONS SUBMITTED BY HON. RICHARD BLUMENTHAL TO ROBERT A. PETZEL, MD, UNDER SECRETARY FOR HEALTH, VETERANS HEALTH ADMINISTRATION (VHA), U.S. DEPARTMENT OF VETERANS AFFAIRS

Question 16. I have heard from one of my constituents that it is difficult for some veterans to obtain their VA Identification Card, which is required to obtain VA health benefits. Can you please provide information about the process a veteran needs to follow and what are the criteria to obtain these benefits?

Response. The Veterans Health Identification Card (VHIC) is for identification and check-in at VA appointments. It cannot be used as a credit card or an insurance card, and it does not authorize or pay for care at non-VA facilities. To receive a VHIC, a Veteran must be enrolled. If the Veteran is not enrolled, the Veteran may apply for enrollment online at www.va.gov/healthbenefits/enroll, by calling 1–877–222–VETS (8387), or apply for enrollment in person at his or her local VA medical facility.

In February 2014, VA began issuing the VHIC to newly enrolled Veterans and enrolled Veterans who were not previously issued the old VIC but requested an identification card. Enrolled Veterans who were not issued the old VIC may contact their local VA medical center Enrollment Coordinator to arrange to have their picture taken for the new VHIC, or they may request a new VHIC at their next VA health care appointment.

Veterans who are already enrolled should ensure the address VA has on file is correct so you can receive your VHIC in a timely manner. For more information, please visit http://www.va.gov/HEALTHBENEFITS/vhic/index.asp.

Chairman SANDERS. Dr. Petzel, thank you very much.
General Coots.

STATEMENT OF BRIGADIER GENERAL NORVELL V. COOTS, USA, DEPUTY COMMANDING GENERAL (SUPPORT), U.S. ARMY MEDICAL COMMAND AND ASSISTANT SURGEON GENERAL FOR FORCE PROJECTION, OFFICE OF THE SURGEON GENERAL, U.S. ARMY; ACCOMPANIED BY COLONEL KEVIN T. GALLOWAY, USA, DIRECTOR, ARMY PAIN MANAGEMENT PROGRAM, REHABILITATION AND REINTEGRATION DIVISION

General COOTS. Chairman Sanders, Ranking Member Burr, and distinguished Members of this Committee, thank you for the opportunity to appear before you to discuss some of the Army Medicine's initiatives to address health and pain management needs of our servicemembers. I am accompanied by Colonel Galloway, who is the director for Army Medicine's Pain Management Program.

On behalf of the over 150,000 dedicated soldiers and civilians that make up Army medicine, I want to extend our appreciation to Congress for the support given to military medicine which provides the resources we need to deliver leading-edge health services to our warriors, families, and retirees.

The Army has been engaged over the last 13 years in combat operations and related activities that have challenged the bodies and spirits of our soldiers and their families. Army medicine has worked with our sister services and the Veterans' Health Administration to meet the emerging medical needs of our servicemembers and veterans.

Our initiatives which are detailed further in my written testimony are aimed at improving outcomes, increasing safety, and enhancing the transition of care to the VA.

Treating pain is one of medicines oldest and more fundamental responsibilities. Yet modern medicine continues to struggle in its efforts to understand pain mechanisms and to relieve pain and suffering of our patients. These complex issues impact patients, providers, leaders, and organizations across the military, the VA, and in the civilian sector. Effective solutions must involve innovative strategies, comprehensive solutions, and collaborative efforts.

While the complicated nature of pain management and overmedication is not unique to the military or military medicine, we do face some unique challenges. We provide medical care on the battlefield and across an 8,000-mile medical evacuation chain that moves injured servicemembers from remote locations to U.S. hospitals with lightening efficiency.

I have been there receiving our wounded warriors during my time in Afghanistan as well as at Walter Reed when I was the hospital commander. I know that for military medical providers, we begin pain management on the battlefield at the point of injury and continue throughout evacuation, treatment, and recovery.

Army medicine initiative aimed at non-opioid medications and regional nerve blocks to provide local relief are important to expanding opioid sparing strategies at the earliest moments of care.

In 2010, the Army-led pain management task force was chartered to develop a comprehensive, holistic, and multi-disciplinary pain management strategy for the DOD. The Army has been working to implement the task force recommendations through the Army pain management campaign and while continuing to build collaborations both inside and outside of the Department of Defense.

Current Army initiatives are aimed at improving pain management, patient care and safety, and reducing adverse outcomes related to prescription drugs. These are all a part of comprehensive strategy that includes establishing a network of standardized pain management capabilities, developing the DOD pain assessment screening tool, and outcomes registry by leveraging previous NIH investment in research, comprehensive medication reviews, and pharmacy screening tools within the medical home which is our primary care model to identify active duty servicemembers at increased risk, expanding the role of clinical pharmacists by embedding them in the medical home as a member of the comprehensive care team, improving pain management specialty support to primary care providers through-out pain ECHO tele-mentoring initiative, expanding our understanding and utilization of effective integrative medicine modalities such as acupuncture, yoga, medical massage, and biofeedback through our collaborative partnerships and collaboration with the National Center for Complementary and Alternative Medicine and the Defense and Veterans' Center for Integrative Pain Management on research studies of non-medication complements or alternatives to standard pain management therapies.

There efforts have been associated with fewer adverse drug-related events, reduced hospital admissions, improved patient outcomes, and overall cost avoidance.

Finally, I would like to mention ongoing work with the VA to endure the smooth transition of care as servicemembers enter the VA system. The overarching pain management task force objective is to provide a standardized DOD and VA approach to optimize the care for warriors and their families.

Our providers and patients benefit from a standardized approach to pain management while they are in uniform and as they transition to the VA health care system.

I want to thank my partners in the DOD, the VA, and our colleagues testifying here today for the efforts made and our shared goals.

I also want to thank Congress and the Committee for your continued support and I look forward to your questions. Army medicine is serving to heal and honored to serve.

[The prepared statement of General Coots follows:]

PREPARED STATEMENT OF BRIGADIER GENERAL NORVELL V. COOTS, DEPUTY COMMANDING GENERAL (SUPPORT), U.S. ARMY MEDICAL COMMAND AND ASSISTANT SURGEON GENERAL FOR FORCE PROJECTION, OFFICE OF THE SURGEON GENERAL, UNITED STATES ARMY AND COLONEL KEVIN T. GALLOWAY, ARMY PAIN MANAGEMENT PROGRAM DIRECTOR, REHABILITATION AND REINTEGRATION DIVISION, OFFICE OF THE SURGEON GENERAL, UNITED STATES ARMY

Chairman Sanders, Ranking Member Burr, and Distinguished Members of this Committee—thank you for the opportunity to appear before you to discuss some of the Army Medicine's initiatives to address healthcare needs of our Soldiers, specifically as they relate to the challenges the entire Nation is facing with pain management and the use of opioids. On behalf of the over 150,000 dedicated Soldiers and civilians that make up Army Medicine, I want to extend our appreciation to Congress for the support given to military medicine, which provides the resources we need to deliver leading edge health services to our Warriors, Families and Retirees. I'm accompanied today by Colonel Kevin Galloway, Director for Army Medicine's Pain Management Program.

The Army has been engaged over the last 13 years in combat operations and related activities that have challenged the bodies and spirits of our Soldiers and their families. Throughout this intensive period of military operations, Army Medicine, along with our Sister Services and the Veterans Health Administration (VHA), have been evolving and adapting to meet the emerging medical needs of our wounded, ill, and injured Servicemembers and Veterans. While some of the medical challenges facing Servicemembers and Veterans are unique to the military and military medicine, the challenges related to pain management and the potential overuse, abuse, and diversion of pain medications are shared by the Nation at large. These complex issues impact patients, providers, leaders and organizations across the military health system, the VHA, and civilian medicine. Consequently, effective solutions and strategies will involve patients, providers, leaders and organizations across military, VHA and civilian medicine. I would like to share some of our innovative strategies, comprehensive solutions, and collaborative efforts with you today as well as emphasize our commitment to continuous improvement and research efforts.

PAIN MANAGEMENT

First, I'd like to place the challenges of pain management in some context. Treating pain is one of medicine's oldest and most fundamental responsibilities, yet modern medicine continues to struggle in its efforts to understand pain mechanisms and to relieve pain and suffering for our patients. Pain is an enigmatic issue for medicine that places significant burdens on patients, families, medical providers, and employers. Pain is the most frequent reason patients seek medical care in the United States. A 2011 Institute of Medicine (IOM) Report noted that more than 116 million Americans suffer from chronic pain. The annual cost of chronic pain in the U.S. is estimated at $560 billion, including health care expenses, lost income, and lost productivity. The Centers for Disease Control identified prescription medication abuse as an ''epidemic'' in the United States. The military is not immune to these challenges.

In 2010, the Army-led Pain Management Task Force was chartered to develop a comprehensive, holistic, multidisciplinary, and multimodal strategy utilizing state-of-the-art/science practices in the field. Comprised of representatives from the Uniformed Services and VHA, the Pain Management Task Force examined staff education, clinical practice, and the structure of pain management in military medicine, the VHA, and in civilian medicine. I would like to emphasize that the Task Force benefited immensely during this analysis from the VHA's previous and ongoing initiatives to develop and implement pain management strategies.

The 2010 Pain Management Task Force Report has been widely circulated and recognized across U.S. Medicine and abroad. The American Academy of Pain Medicine recognized the Pain Management Task Force with its Presidential Commendation. One year after the release of the report, the IOM released its own report entitled, ''Relieving Pain in America,'' which acknowledged and referenced the work of the Pain Management Task Force. More importantly, the IOM report's findings and recommendations largely paralleled those contained in the Pain Management Task Force Report. When the IOM report was released in June 2011, the Army was already operationalizing the Pain Management Task Force's recommendations through the Comprehensive Pain Management Campaign Plan. Since the release of the IOM report, the Army has been representing the Department of Defense on the National Institutes of Health (NIH) Interagency Pain Research Coordinating Committee, the Federal advisory committee created by the Department of Health and Human Services to enhance pain research efforts and promote collaboration across the government.

The Comprehensive Pain Management Campaign Plan provides a roadmap for this holistic, multimodal, multidisciplinary pain management strategy. Army Medicine's pain strategy includes several lines of effort: first, to implement a culture of pain awareness, education, and proactive intervention; second, to provide tools and infrastructure that support and encourage practice and research advancements in pain management; and last, to build a full spectrum of best practices for the continuum of acute and chronic pain, based on a foundation of the best available medical evidence.

The foundation of the MEDCOM pain management program is developing a tiered or ''Stepped Care'' strategy that provides the appropriate level of pain management capability, provider education and access to consultative/referral support at each level of care (i.e. from Primary Care to Specialty Care). Interdisciplinary Pain Management Centers (IPMC) are being established at each of the Army's eight medical centers. IPMCs provide the highest tier of pain management delivered by a multidisciplinary team of providers working together to provide consultation, care, and expertise for interventional pain medicine. Our goals are rehabilitation and functional restoration through these integrative medicine modalities.

The Army Pain Management Extension for Community Healthcare Outcomes (ECHO) tele-mentoring initiative leverages the model developed by the University of New Mexico (UNM) Project ECHO initiative. The Army is completing a two-year collaboration with UNM to adapt this best practice for use in the Army's pain program. ECHO's objective is to complement the capacity, competence and confidence of remote primary care providers. Utilizing weekly video teleconferencing to create regional communities of practice, ECHO links the IPMC specialty teams (i.e. hubs) with their designated Patient Centered Medical Homes (i.e. spokes). This improves provider knowledge, increases care coordination, and decreases the need for continued specialty referrals to the direct and purchased care systems.

28

COMPLEMENTARY INTEGRATIVE MEDICINE MODALITIES

As recommended by the Pain Management Task Force, the integrative medicine modalities in our IPMCs include acupuncture, movement therapy/yoga, medical massage, and bio-feedback. The use of these modalities in our IPMCs provides our patients with non-medication pain management options. The Army has been collaborating with several organizations with a common interest in expanding the utilization of complementary integrative medicine modalities. The National Center for Complementary and Alternative Medicine at NIH, the Bravewell Collaborative, and the Samueli Institute have all been extremely helpful in this effort.

Army clinicians are participating with the Air Force, Navy, and VHA in a $5.4 million Joint Incentive Fund Project to field a standardized basic acupuncture training and sustainment model across DOD and VHA medical facilities. Training teams have already started traveling to Army, Navy, Air Force, and VHA medical facilities to deliver this training. The response from providers and patients has been overwhelmingly positive.

Army Medicine, along with the Navy and Air Force, is collaborating through the Defense and Vet Center for Integrative Pain Management on research studies related to the use of acupuncture and yoga as non-medication complements/alternatives to standard pain management therapies. Initial evidence indicates these can be effective complements and sometimes an alternative to medications.

PAIN OUTCOMES MEASUREMENT

In response to the 2010 National Defense Authorization Act and the recommendations in the Pain Management Task Force Report, the DOD began development of the Pain Assessment Screening Tool and Outcomes Registry (PASTOR). PASTOR was designed as a tool to reduce the burden of questionnaires during clinical contact through modern information technology, make use of well-established pain assessment tools already available, and provide a framework for development of new assessment tools. Furthermore, PASTOR is envisioned as a critical first step in realizing the vision of outcomes driven pain care across the DOD and VHA health care systems.

The PASTOR prototype results in a clinician report, displaying alerts for concerning responses to questions covering PTSD, depression, anxiety, and alcohol use. These alerts are intended to prompt further individualized evaluation by the clinician. Areas of greatest pain are mapped on an image of a body, and self-reported pain values are tracked over time. When these scores are analyzed in concert with validated measures of emotional (anxiety, depression, anger) and physical (sleep, physical function) health domains, trends are easily identified. Additionally, each patient has an opportunity to list and rate ability on activities that are important to that individual. This functional data provides practical indicators of pain management success. A new set of opioid use measures are also under development and will be field tested in both civilian and military setting later this year.

A significant advantage in the PASTOR development program is its collaborative partnership and development strategy with the NIH Patient Reported Outcomes Measurement Information Systems, or PROMIS. PROMIS represents an existing Federal investment of approximately $100 million, over 8 years of research and development, and the product of 150 scientists at 15 primary research sites. PROMIS created more than 80 royalty free instruments which can be used to capture numerous components of health related quality of life including physical health, mental health and social health. Computerized adaptive testing (CAT)—enables computer-based delivery of measures which can obtain clinical accuracy in five items or less. Scientists at Northwestern University have teamed with the military to integrate brief PROMIS measures with the needs of military personnel and their families who require pain management. This reduction in patient burden, without loss of clinical reliability, enables PASTOR to frequently assess multiple facets of pain and opioid use.

Thus far, a working prototype has been constructed, pain threshold values for appropriate initiation of PASTOR have been identified, and a pilot test of the system has begun in two military treatment facilities, with more to follow in the coming months.

Army Medicine is adopting the Defense and Veterans Pain Rating Scale (DVPRS). Something as simple as changing how we ask our patients about their pain can impact the prevalence of medication use. The scale was developed by the Pain Management Task Force and validated through DOD/VHA research studies. It recalibrates the pain discussion along the lines of: ``How is pain affecting your function and quality of life?'' The scale includes supplemental questions on pain's effect on sleep, mood, stress and activity. The Army is integrating DVPRS into the Patient Centered Medical Home workflows.

Another area I'd like to highlight with regard to pain management is our ongoing collaboration with the VHA to ensure the smooth transition of care for Soldiers who will be receiving care in the VHA health system. Prominently positioned on the Pain Management Task Force Report cover is the overarching Task Force objective: "Providing a standardized DOD and VHA vision and approach to pain management to optimize the care for Warriors and their Families." Army Medicine has continued to engage with the Air Force, Navy and VHA to move our organizations in that direction. The Army Pain Management Program's incorporation of the VHA's Stepped Care approach synchronizes provider education with the expectations of our patients. Not only do our military providers and patients benefit from a standardized approach to pain management while they are in uniform, but this also makes the transition to VHA care far less disruptive.

DOD and VHA collaboration has also resulted in standardized prescription medication formularies to ensure Soldiers with chronic pain are able to continue effective care plans after their transition to the VHA. Last, military and VHA providers are engaged in a project to develop and implement a common pain management education curriculum for both providers and patients. The curriculum will be fully developed within the next twelve months, and will be implemented across VHA and DOD within the next eighteen months. These initiatives will take us closer to the standardized DOD and VHA vision and approach to pain management referenced by the Pain Task Force.

In addition to the Pain Management Campaign, Army Medicine is addressing the potential overuse, abuse and diversion of opioids through a comprehensive strategy that integrates several other initiatives including Polypharmacy, Substance Abuse, Behavioral Health, and Warrior Transition Care.

Soldiers with complex injuries often require the use of multiple medications (i.e. polypharmacy) which can place them at greater risk for medication-related adverse events. The Army seeks to reduce risk, enhance safety and optimize care by including the Soldier, Family members, healthcare providers, pharmacists and commanders as part of the healthcare team. Army policies also establish procedures to identify polypharmacy trends that could lead to misuse by Soldiers and Wounded Warriors.

Army Medicine uses best practices that are comparable to, or exceed, civilian programs, such as prescription drug monitoring to identify polypharmacy cases. Positive interventions include comprehensive medication reviews, sole provider programs, limiting the dispensed supply of medication, restricting high-risk patients to the utilization of one pharmacy, informed consent, use of non-drug treatment options, clinical pharmacist referrals, and patient and provider education.

The Army trains its providers on the risks of prescription opioid overuse and ways to prevent medication misuse. The US Army Public Health Command and the Uniformed Services University of the Health Sciences developed an interactive storyline-based training aimed at increasing the knowledge and skills health professionals need to better interact with Soldiers in a clinic setting. Army Medicine has implemented systems and procedures our clinicians regularly use to prevent and detect issues of opioid overuse. These tools include the ability for our clinicians to review all prescriptions paid for by the Defense Health Agency (DHA) pharmacy benefit regardless of the point of service (Military, Home Delivery or Retail Pharmacy). The DHA Pharmacoeconomic Branch Web site allows clinicians to identify concerning use of opioids dispensed under the TRICARE Pharmacy Benefit through the use of prescription screening tools such as the Medication Analysis and Reporting Tools.

Army Medicine is expanding the role of clinical pharmacists to address national concerns with polypharmacy and adverse drug events that lead to hospital admissions. The Army Surgeon General supports evidence-based enhancements drawing on the expertise and contributions of pharmacists embedded in Patient-Centered Medical Homes. The addition of clinical pharmacists to the patient care team translates into decreased overall costs, fewer adverse drug-related events, reduced hospital admissions, and improved medication-related patient outcomes and appropriate adherence to medications. Clinical pharmacists improve readiness of the force through policy and practice, systematically identifying Soldiers with polypharmacy risk and communicating these concerns to health care providers. The Army uses an automated polypharmacy screening tool to screen all Active Duty Servicemembers monthly to identify Soldiers prescribed different combinations of high risk medications. These reports are provided to the medical team for review and follow-up. Clinical pharmacists embedded in Army medical homes optimize patient adherence to appropriate drug therapy by conducting medication reviews, resolving medication problems and recommending cost effective treatment alternatives.

Current Army initiatives aimed at reducing adverse outcomes and harm due to prescription drug abuses include informed consent for polypharmacy, sole provider program, limiting authorized use of prescriptions to six months following the prescription fill date, adjusting the panel of drugs in random urine drug testing to include prescription drugs and polypharmacy education for healthcare providers and patients.

Healthcare providers must review identified risks and potential interactions with the Soldier, provide education on detection and management of interactions, and must document informed consent in the medical record. Informed consent includes a brief description of discussed risks and whether or not the indication for which the medication is being used is a Food and Drug Administration (FDA) approved indication or the medication is used off-label.

The Army policy instructs healthcare providers to have a low threshold for referring patients to Behavioral Health resources and the Sole Prescriber Program. Healthcare providers enroll Soldiers at increased risk of adverse effects, drug interactions, or inappropriate medication use in the Sole Prescriber Program to optimize care. Once enrolled, only a Soldier's designated provider or alternate provider is authorized to prescribe controlled substances for the Soldier. If necessary, the Soldier may be restricted to a specific pharmacy or pharmacies by activating the Prescription Lock-out Program.

In addition to Soldiers who are identified as having intentional or unintentional risk for medication overdose, healthcare providers will refer Soldiers who present with polypharmacy-related concerns to a clinical pharmacist. The pharmacist will identify medication-related problems, develop a medication action plan, and provide medication education to the patient. Clinical pharmacists document patient encounters and consultations for medication therapy management in an electronic medical record template to improve communication with providers.

Army policy limits authorized use of prescriptions to six months following the prescription fill date. In addition, Army medical providers may prescribe only the minimum quantity of controlled substances necessary to treat an acute illness or injury, and quantities of controlled substances used to treat acute conditions are dispensed as a 30-day supply. Prescribers and pharmacists inform Soldiers that, per Army policy, controlled substance prescriptions have an expiration date of six months from the dispensed date, and that a positive urinalysis test for the drug after six months from dispensing may result in a "no legitimate use" finding.

Polypharmacy education and training is available to healthcare providers and beneficiaries to improve appropriate prescribing and use of medications, respectively. Patient-specific training is available to Warrior Transition Units (WTU) to improve awareness of safe medication use, proper medication disposal, and promotion for the bi-annual drug take back events.

Army Medicine has participated in all Drug Enforcement Agency (DEA) National Prescription Drug Take Back Day events since their inception in 2010. Thirty-six Army Military Treatment Facilities participated in the Take Back Day on 25 and 26 October 2013, with over 2,000 patients participating and 7,491 pounds of unused medications collected. The Army will continue to participate in bi-annual Take Back events in an effort to maintain attention on the importance of appropriate disposal of medications that are no longer needed. Army Medicine provides support through coordinated public affairs communications and education directed at medical staff, patients, Families and military leadership, to include on-site presence at every designated event.

SUBSTANCE ABUSE PROGRAMS

The Army continues to synchronize clinical care and processes provided through the Army Substance Abuse Program and Army Medical Command's primary care providers, pain specialists, and behavioral health specialists. The Army uses the DOD's drug testing program to test not only for illegal drugs, but also for prescribed medications taken inappropriately (that is without an active prescription). Identified Soldiers are referred to the Army Substance Abuse Program where they are assessed and enrolled for treatment. Commanders and clinicians support this treatment process regardless of the Soldier's disposition, because we recognize that we have an obligation to ensure our Soldiers remain effective on active duty or make their transition from active service with drug use properly managed.

BEHAVIORAL HEALTH PROGRAM

Army Medicine's Behavioral Health Service Line is an interconnected group of standardized programs delivering a wide variety of Behavioral Health services to Soldiers and beneficiaries. For the treatment of substance abuse disorders, the Army has five Addiction Medicine Intensive Outpatient Programs. There are currently 187 beds designated for long-term Substance Use Disorder treatment in the Military Health System, 22 of which are in the Army. These Military Health System facilities have consistently had 85% or higher utilization rates for the past 18 months. Purchased care inpatient substance use disorder treatment accounts for approximately 70 Soldiers per month. Demand for network inpatient substance use disorder treatment has decreased sharply with the implementation of the NDAA 2010, Section 596, but continues to remain high enough to justify increases in capacity in the coming years to recapture inpatient substance use disorder care going to the network.

Army Medical Command conducted an analysis of all health care and pharmacy records involving Army Active Duty Servicemembers, reflecting an annual average population of 657,000 Soldiers from 2007 to 2012. This analysis showed a 65% increase in the number of Soldiers seeking behavioral health services (151,620 in 2007 to 250,410 in 2012), and a corresponding 44% increase in the number of Soldiers prescribed any medication within the broad psychiatric category (101,914 in 2007 to 147,197 in 2012). In other words, there has not been any disproportionate increase in medication use. There are multiple safeguards in place to ensure that psychiatric medications, including antipsychotic medications, are prescribed safely and judiciously according to accepted clinical practice guidelines and nationally recognized standards of care.

MEDICAL HOME AND WARRIOR TRANSITION CLINICS

Optimizing the use of medications through pharmacist interaction as part of a Patient Centered Care Team is best exemplified by their work within the Wounded Warrior Clinics. Of the 22 Warrior Clinics in support of Army Medicine Warrior Transition Units, 21 Clinics are currently supported by approximately 25 clinical pharmacists and 5 pharmacy technicians. These Warrior Clinics are consistent with the Medical Home model, where pharmacists manage complex medication regimens and mitigate risks for Wounded Warriors.

The Risk Assessment Management within the Warrior Care and Transition Program enables WTUs to monitor the safety of Soldiers. WTU Commanders, in coordination with the Soldiers' interdisciplinary team, conduct risk assessments for every Soldier. The initial risk assessment occurs within 24 hours of the Soldier's arrival at the WTU, ongoing assessments are regularly made throughout the Soldier's stay, and additional assessments occur during key events such as during quarterly scrimmages as directed by the Soldier's personalized Comprehensive Training Plan. Risk assessments focus on therapy adherence, behavioral health history, substance abuse history, and access to care patterns. The intent is to assess whether Soldiers on these medications need additional monitoring and assistance with medication management. If a Soldier is identified as needing additional monitoring and assistance, the interdisciplinary team determines what risk mitigation strategies are needed to maintain the Soldier's safety. If needed, the Soldier is entered into the Army Medical Department's Sole Provider Program. Soldiers enrolled in the Sole Provider Program may only receive medications from their assigned provider, and receive no more than a 7-day supply of narcotics or psychotropic medications. Clinical Pharmacists also provide oversight as they review the medication profiles of all Soldiers in a WTU, who are determined to be at high risk. These reviews occur at least weekly.

Army Medicine has engaged in a comprehensive campaign to address the pain management needs of Soldiers and their Families. Our strategy involves developing and implementing solutions with our DOD, VHA, and Civilian Medicine partners. Thank you again for the opportunity to testify before the Committee and for your support to our Soldiers and Veterans.

RESPONSE TO POSTHEARING QUESTIONS SUBMITTED BY HON. BERNARD SANDERS TO BG NORVELL V. COOTS, USA, DEPUTY COMMANDING GENERAL (SUPPORT), U.S. ARMY MEDICAL COMMAND AND ASSISTANT SURGEON GENERAL FOR FORCE PROJECTION, OFFICE OF THE SURGEON GENERAL, U.S. ARMY

COMPLEMENTARY AND ALTERNATIVE MEDICINE (CAM)

Question 1. How can the Army improve access to CAM therapies among servicemembers? How can it help improve what information is available to servicemembers and their providers about CAM services?

Response. In Army Medicine, perhaps the single greatest application of Complementary and Alternative Medicine (CAM) has been seen in pain management. Initially, Servicemembers were often the ones who identified integrative medicine treatments to their medical providers as uniquely effective in restoring and maintaining their health with minimal side effects. In response to this call to action and as a result of increasing medical evidence, Army Medicine has deliberately expanded its experience and utilization with integrative medicine as part of the Army's Comprehensive Pain Management Program.

The Army Pain Program has been moving toward a more multi-disciplinary, multimodal pain management strategy that leverages selected CAM modalities alongside more conventional pain management treatments such as medications and interventional procedures such as injections, nerve blocks, and surgeries. In addition to chiropractic care, the Army's Interdisciplinary Pain Management Centers are employing modalities such as acupuncture, massage therapy, movement therapies to include yoga, and biofeedback. These are all proving to be effective complements and sometimes alternatives to medications.

Army Medicine will continue to expand the utilization and collection of evidence regarding the efficacy of integrative medicine modalities alongside more conventional therapies.

Question 2. What factors currently limit DOD from further broadening CAM therapies across the Army and other branches?

Response. Of the many treatment strategies addressed in the Army's Comprehensive Pain Management Campaign Plan, the use of CAM therapies has been one of the most challenging. As noted in the Army's 2010 Pain Task Force Report, there are an increasing number of reports in medical literature regarding the safety and efficacy of these treatment modalities, and their use is becoming more widespread across medicine. It is believed that the use of the various CAM modalities can lead to an improved sense of being, health status or functional outcome through pain reduction, lower medication usage or increased quality of life. However, there is still a paucity of evidence-based scientific literature on the precise role for these modalities in the overall management of acute and chronic pain.

Per the Code of Federal Regulations, Section 199.4(g)(15), TRICARE is unable to pay for healthcare in the purchased care sector that has not been proven to be both safe and effective in the treatment of the underlying condition. While there have been an increasing number of articles published on the use of CAM for the treatment of acute and chronic pain, there have been no evidence-based clinical practice guidelines published or other evidence based protocols developed that incorporate the general use of CAM, or specific types of CAM.

However, within the DOD, Military Treatment Facilities (MTFs) are allowed, under very specific conditions and specifications, to offer certain types of services that would otherwise not be covered benefits under TRICARE. That is the case with certain CAM therapies. Under these circumstances, the MTF Commander is responsible for ensuring that all existing community standards of care are met, to include any credentialing requirements of practitioners if they are not otherwise considered to be TRICARE authorized providers. Army Medicine is working with the Navy and Air Force to develop credentialing guidelines and oversight provisions to provide appropriate, standardized credentialing of practitioners who will employ CAM at our MTFs.

One notable exception can be seen in the military's expanded use of chiropractic care. Unlike the other CAM modalities, chiropractic care was originally offered in 1995 as a demonstration program and later expanded as directed under Section 702 of the National Defense Authorization Act (NDAA) for Fiscal Year 2001. Three subsequent NDAA's allowed for expansion of the program, resulting in chiropractic services now being offered at 62 MTFs but still limited to Active Duty Servicemembers.

ACUPUNCTURE TRAINING

Question 3. How would the Joint Incentive Fund Project to implement a standardized acupuncture training and sustainment model across DOD and VA medical facilities improve acupuncture services the Army provides servicemembers? When can we expect system-wide implementation of this joint model?

Response. The variances in acupuncture integration, utilization, reimbursement, and practice in health systems are not limited to Federal/military medicine. The absence of universally accepted protocols, credentialing, and clinical practice guidelines have inhibited more aggressive implementation across the DOD and VHA health systems. The $5.4 million, Joint Incentive Fund (JIF) acupuncture project will develop, pilot, evaluate and implement a uniform tiered acupuncture education and training program for Military Health System (MHS) and Veterans Health Administration (VHA) providers in order to provide initial and expanded access to this modality across MHS and VHA treatment facilities.

The acupuncture JIF provides a pathway to uniform implementation and integration of this modality across military and VA healthcare systems through a proven practical program of training and certification for providers. It drives adoption and further development of acupuncture best practices across the MHS and VHA. The two-year acupuncture JIF project is scheduled to be completed by 2016. In progress reviews are provided to the Health Executive Council on a quarterly basis.

Question 4. How many providers trained in acupuncture already working in the Army? How many of these providers exclusively offer acupuncture services? On average, how many hours per week do these offer acupuncture to servicemembers?

Response. U.S. Army Medical Command (MEDCOM) providers, including physicians, physician assistants, nurse practitioners and dentists who wish to use acupuncture in their practice are required to document their acupuncture training and competency in their facility credentialing file. As of April 2014, 46 MEDCOM providers have added acupuncture to their credentialing files. None of these providers are exclusively offering acupuncture services but use acupuncture as a complementary modality in their practice.

The number of hours per week where acupuncture is offered is not possible to calculate. However, the Army does capture the number of acupuncture procedure performance. In FY 2012, over 23,000 acupuncture procedures were performed in Army medical treatment facilities. The FY 2013 numbers for acupuncture utilization is currently unavailable but should trend upwards.

The Army pain management program has been working to integrate licensed acupuncturists in the eight Army interdisciplinary pain management clinics. These individuals are being hired with a primary responsibility to provide acupuncture. At this time, the Army Pain Program, along with the Air Force, Navy, and VHA are working to standardize coding, treatment protocols, and credentialing for licensed acupuncturists.

Question 5. Is the current amount of acupuncture offered within the Army sufficient to meet the demand for this therapy? If not, what efforts are being made to ensure an adequate number are available to treat veterans once the joint model is implemented?

Response. The current capacity within the Army direct healthcare system is insufficient to support the perceived demand for acupuncture.

While the Joint Incentive Fund acupuncture project to field a standardized basic acupuncture training and sustainment model across DOD and VHA will greatly improve access to basic acupuncture techniques, there will likely be a need for additional organized efforts to increase the enterprise wide training, availability, and utilization of acupuncture and other complementary integrative modalities.

DOD/VA COLLABORATION

Question 6. What benefits has DOD seen from the standardization of the prescription medication between VA and DOD available to both servicemembers and veterans? Are servicemembers able to continue their existing course of treatment as they transition to VA health care?

Response. Ongoing efforts to harmonize formularies are aimed at improving continuity of care for DOD beneficiaries transitioning to the VA. The VA has established policy that supports the continuation of DOD prescribed medications upon transfer whether or not the drug is listed on the formulary or if its use is consistent with VA prescribing guidelines. The VA provider is permitted to change previously prescribed medications to allow consistency with prescribing guidelines after careful consideration and implementation to prevent avoidable problems.

Question 7. What other efforts have DOD and VA taken to collaborate and stand-ardize treatment options available to servicemembers and veterans for chronic pain?

Response. Phased implementation of the Comprehensive Pain Management Campaign Plan is ongoing across Army Medicine and Tri-Service/VA implementation of Task Force recommendations continues as part of Health Executive Council Pain Management Work Group. In FY 2013, Army, Air Force, Navy, and the VA demonstrated increased interest and activity in synchronized implementation of Pain Task Force Recommendations. Uniformed Services and the VA will focus on executing several joint pain management projects as listed below. These projects will provide information to Defense Health Agency and Uniformed Services in order to facilitate re-evaluation and possible revisions of policies.

  a. Pain Management Outcome Tool
  b. Tiered Acupuncture Course for Primary Care Providers
  c. Development/Implementation of DOD/VHA education curriculum
  d. Synchronized DOD/VA transition policies for medications

One specific project that highlights DOD/VA collaboration is the basic acupuncture training course. Army clinicians are participating with the Air Force, Navy, and VHA in a $5.4M Joint Incentive Fund Project to field a standardized basic acupuncture training and sustainment model across DOD and VHA medical facilities. Training teams have already started traveling to Army, Navy, Air Force, and VHA medical facilities to deliver this training. The response from providers and patients has been overwhelmingly positive.

————

RESPONSE TO POSTHEARING QUESTIONS SUBMITTED BY HON. RICHARD BLUMENTHAL TO BG NORVELL V. COOTS, USA, DEPUTY COMMANDING GENERAL (SUPPORT), U.S. ARMY MEDICAL COMMAND AND ASSISTANT SURGEON GENERAL FOR FORCE PROJECTION, OFFICE OF THE SURGEON GENERAL, U.S. ARMY

Question 8. Do you have any further breakdown as to the usage for each of the branches of the Armed Forces?

Response. Yes. Information is available on the usage of opiates for all branches of the Armed Forces. Question #9 and #10 responses provide information for Army Servicemembers.

Question 9. How much of the opioid use is for acute conditions and for chronic conditions?

Response. For acute conditions, the proportion of Active Duty Army Servicemembers prescribed an opiate medication at least once in a year for the last 10 years is as follows:

      2004—21%
      2005—22%
      2006—25%
      2007—26%
      2008—26%
      2009—26%
      2010—27%
      2011—29%
      2012—29%
      2013—27%

Chronic opioid use is defined as cumulative use of 90 or greater days of use in a six-month period. Information on chronic use is provided in the response to question #10.

Question 10. How much opioid use is for >90 days in duration?

Response. Chronic opioid use is defined as cumulative use of 90 or greater days of use in a six-month period. The proportion of Active Duty Army Servicemembers with any chronic opiate use in a year is as follows:

      2004—1.27%
      2005—1.54%
      2006—1.76%
      2007—1.96%
      2008—1.95%
      2009—1.97%
      2010—2.09%
      2011—2.36%
      2012—2.57%
      2013—2.34%

RESPONSE TO POSTHEARING QUESTIONS SUBMITTED BY HON. MARK BEGICH TO BG NORVELL V. COOTS, USA, DEPUTY COMMANDING GENERAL (SUPPORT), U.S. ARMY MEDICAL COMMAND AND ASSISTANT SURGEON GENERAL FOR FORCE PROJECTION, OFFICE OF THE SURGEON GENERAL, U.S. ARMY

Question 11. PTSD, depression, TBI, family stress, disability, and joblessness plague our veterans' community and increase the risk of our veterans overmedicating to soothe chronic pain. How are you addressing growing mental health issues in conjunction with pain management? How does this initiative take into account rural and remote locations that may not have Behavioral Health professionals or telehealth?

Response. In the past several years, the Army has vastly expanded and completely overhauled its system of behavioral healthcare and pain management program to address complex co-morbidities and co-occurring conditions.. The Army's Behavioral Health Service Line is comprised of 11 interconnected standardized programs that provide consistent and ready access to behavioral health services covering all behavioral health conditions across our supported beneficiary population.

The 2010 Army-led Pain Management Task Force was chartered to develop a strategy that is comprehensive, holistic, multidisciplinary, and multimodal, utilizing state-of-the-art/science practices in the field resulting in the Comprehensive Pain Management Campaign Plan. Army Medicine's pain strategy includes three primary lines of effort: 1) implement a culture of pain awareness, education, and proactive intervention, 2) provide tools and infrastructure that support and encourage practice and research advancements in pain management, and 3) build a full spectrum of best practices for the continuum of acute and chronic pain, based on a foundation of the best available medical evidence. This includes incorporating behavioral health care as part of pain management solutions and ensuring pain management for Soldiers and pain management training for providers outside of the main area of care.

Soldiers with complex injuries often require polypharmacy, or the use of multiple medications, which place them at greater risk for medication-related adverse events. The Army seeks to reduce risk, enhance safety and optimize care by including the Soldier, Family members, healthcare providers, pharmacists and commanders as part of the healthcare team. Army policies establish procedures to identify polypharmacy trends that could lead to misuse by Soldiers and Wounded Warriors.

Army Medicine also uses best practices that are comparable to, or exceed, civilian programs, such as prescription drug monitoring to identify polypharmacy cases. Positive interventions include comprehensive medication reviews, sole provider programs, limiting the dispensed supply of medication, restricting high-risk patients to the utilization of one pharmacy, informed consent, use of non-drug treatment options, clinical pharmacist referrals, and patient and provider education.

The Army trains its providers on the risks of prescription opioid overuse and ways to prevent medication misuse. Army Medicine has implemented systems and procedures our clinicians regularly use to prevent and detect issues of opioid overuse. These tools include the ability for our clinicians to review all prescriptions paid for by the Defense Health Agency (DHA) pharmacy benefit regardless of the point of service (Military, Home Delivery or Retail Pharmacy).

The Army policy instructs healthcare providers to have a low threshold for referring patients to Behavioral Health resources and the Sole Prescriber Program. Healthcare providers enroll Soldiers at increased risk of adverse effects, drug interactions, or inappropriate medication use in the Sole Prescriber Program to optimize care. Once enrolled, only a Soldier's designated provider or alternate provider is authorized to prescribe controlled substances for the Soldier. If necessary, the Soldier may be restricted to a specific pharmacy or pharmacies by activating the Prescription Lock-out Program.

In addition to Soldiers who are identified as having intentional or unintentional risk for medication overdose, healthcare providers will refer Soldiers who present with polypharmacy-related concerns to a clinical pharmacist.

Army Medicine is expanding the role of clinical pharmacists to address national concerns with polypharmacy and adverse drug events that lead to hospital admissions. The Army Surgeon General supports evidence-based enhancements drawing on the expertise and contributions of pharmacists embedded in Patient-Centered Medical Homes.

Army Medicine has participated in all Drug Enforcement Agency (DEA) National Prescription Drug Take Back Day events since their inception in 2010. Thirty-six Army Military Treatment Facilities participated in the Take Back Day on 25 and 26 October 2013, with over 2,000 patients participating and 7,491 pounds of unused medications collected. The Army will continue to participate in bi-annual Take Back events in an effort to maintain attention on the importance of appropriate disposal of medications that are no longer needed. Army Medicine provides support through coordinated public affairs communications and education directed at medical staff, patients, Families and military leadership, to include on-site presence at every designated event.

Specific to Telehealth, the Army has developed and vastly expanded a comprehensive Telehealth system over the past several years that now enables the Army to cross-level clinical care capacity across the globe. In fiscal year 2013, Army clinicians offered care across 18 time zones and in over 30 countries and territories, to include remote locations where Soldiers serve. In fiscal year 2013, Army clinicians provided over 34,000 patient encounters and provider-to-provider tele-consultations in garrison; approximately 85 percent of these encounters were related to outreach via Tele-Behavioral Health.

The Army's Pain Management Task Force recommended the Army "Expand telemedicine capabilities to incorporate pain management initiatives" (Pain Management Task Force, 2010). The Army Pain Management Extension for Community Healthcare Outcomes (ECHO) tele-mentoring initiative leverages the model developed by the University of New Mexico (UNM) Project ECHO initiative. The Army is completing a two-year collaboration with UNM to adapt this best practice for use in the Army's pain program. ECHO's objective is to complement the capacity, competence and confidence of remote primary care providers. Utilizing weekly video tele-conferencing to create regional communities of practice, ECHO links the IPMC specialty teams (i.e. hubs) with their designated Patient Centered Medical Homes (i.e. spokes). This improves provider knowledge, increases care coordination, and decreases the need for continued specialty referrals to the direct and purchased care systems. Army Pain ECHO will be available to Providers supporting Community Based Warrior Transition Units (CBWTU). Additionally, the Army is collaborating with the Air Force, Navy, and Veterans Health Administration on development and utilization of a common DOD/VHA Pain ECHO education curriculum.

Chairman SANDERS. General Coots, thank you very much.
Dr. Briggs.

STATEMENT OF JOSEPHINE BRIGGS, M.D., DIRECTOR, NATIONAL CENTER FOR COMPLEMENTARY AND ALTERNATIVE MEDICINE, NATIONAL INSTITUTES OF HEALTH

Dr. BRIGGS. Good morning, Chairman Sanders, Ranking Member Burr, and Members of the Committee. I want to add my well wishes to Senator Boozman.

Thank you very much for inviting me. I am the Director of the National Center for Complementary and Alternative Medicine at the National Institutes of Health. NCCAM is the leading Federal agency responsible for research on the usefulness and safety of complementary and integrative health practices.

The most common reason Americans turn to these health approaches is for treatment of pain. Pain is a major health problem affecting over 100 million Americans. It is one of the main drivers of our horrific national epidemic of prescription drug abuse.

As a physician, I am well aware that drugs, including opioids, are absolutely essential for the management of pain but also of their serious side effects including overmedication dependency and even death.

As a Nation, we need to find the appropriate balance between the substantial benefits of these medications and the risks. Deaths from opioids exceed those attributed to cocaine and heroin combined. Every day over 100 Americans die of drug overdoses, mostly from prescription painkillers.

Opioids are particularly deadly when combined with Post Traumatic Stress Disorder; and as this Committee knows well, pain and PTSD is a common and tough combination faced by many veterans, also a very common problem in civilian populations. So, finding better alternatives for pain management is an absolutely critical national need.

Concern about research on better strategies for pain management is shared by leadership across the NIH. I serve as one of the co-directors of the Trans-NIH Pain Consortium and a member of the Federal Interagency Pain Research Coordinating Committee. Together with other Federal leaders, we are partnering to develop a cooperative research strategy to meet these important needs.

Some of the very active areas of NIH research include the development of better pain measures including some of the measures that have been incorporated by the DOD, the PASTOR PROMIS measures, for example, understanding why acute pain sometimes turns into chronic pain, and the development of pain medications with less abuse potential.

NCCAM's particular focus is strengthening non-pharmacological treatment and self-management of pain. The evidence that some complementary approaches are of value in pain management is reflected in evidence-based guidelines from the American College of Physicians and the American Pain Society.

Select practices including meditation, acupuncture, spinal manipulation, massage, and hypnosis are increasingly part of the kind of integrative care being offered in some of our health care settings, including hospitals, nursing homes, hospices, and most notably, health facilities in the Veterans' Administration and Department of Defense.

Integrative practitioners place particular emphasis on a patient-centered approach that identifies patient goals and, when appropriate, minimizes the use of drugs.

Research on the mechanism and efficacy and safety of these approaches is the highest priority for NCCAM. We hope to learn how they work, who they help, and how they can be strengthened to better help people with chronic pain.

As part of this effort, we have established a new intramural program that will study the biologic underpinnings of pain using state-of-the-art neuroscience methods to study the brain.

We are particularly delighted to be embarking on an important partnership with the DOD and VA to support the value of these approaches to address the needs of military personnel and veterans for improvement non-pharmacological management of pain together with conditions such as PTSD, depression, and anxiety.

We are funding new studies in partnership with the DOD, VA, National Institute on Drug Abuse, and the National Institute on Alcohol Abuse and Alcoholism on these important problems.

We have created a working group of members of NCCAM's advisory council to advise us on this research agenda. The working group includes distinguished DOD and VA officials such as former Army Surgeon General Eric Schoomaker and the VA's Dr. Tracy Gaudet. It is chaired by Dr. Lloyd Michener, Director of Family Medicine at Duke University.

In summary, Mr. Chairman, NIH and NCCAM are committed to partnerships with the VA and the DOD to strengthen research to understand pain, to improve pain management, and reduce over-medication and opioid dependency.

Thank you. I am very happy to be here and happy to answer any questions.

[The prepared statement of Dr. Briggs follows:]

PREPARED STATEMENT OF JOSEPHINE BRIGGS, M.D., DIRECTOR, NATIONAL CENTER FOR COMPLEMENTARY AND ALTERNATIVE MEDICINE, NATIONAL INSTITUTES OF HEALTH, U.S. DEPARTMENT OF HEALTH AND HUMAN SERVICES

Chairman Sanders, Ranking Member Burr, and Members of the Committee, thank you for inviting me to be here today to discuss the need to improve pain management strategies to reduce overmedication and opioid dependency. My name is Josephine Briggs, M.D., and I am the Director of the National Center for Complementary and Alternative Medicine (NCCAM) at the National Institutes of Health (NIH), the Federal Government's lead agency for supporting scientific research on complementary practices and integrative health interventions. Our mission at NCCAM is to define the usefulness and safety of complementary and integrative health practices and their role in improving health through rigorous scientific investigation. Our research priorities are driven by scientific promise and public health need. We support the study of complementary interventions, approaches, and disciplines across the continuum of basic, translational, efficacy, and effectiveness research.

Complementary, alternative, and integrative health practices are defined as having origins outside of mainstream conventional medicine. They include both self-care practices like meditation, yoga, and dietary supplements, and health care provider administered care such as acupuncture, and chiropractic, osteopathic, and naturopathic medicine. As these modalities are increasingly integrated into mainstream health care, NCCAM is committed to developing the evidence needed by the public, health care professionals, and policymakers to make informed decisions about their use and integration into medical practice. In addition to supporting the research, we disseminate the latest evidence-based information on these approaches to scientists, health care providers, and the general public through an information-rich Web site (www.nccam.nih.gov) and other media.

According to the Centers for Disease Control and Prevention, approximately 30 percent to 40 percent of Americans use complementary and integrative health practices, spending some $34 billion in 2007.[1] This represents 1.5 percent of total health expenditures and 11 percent of out-of-pocket costs. These practices are increasingly being offered in hospitals and hospice settings. The most common reason cited for use of complementary and integrative health practices is for the alleviation of pain.

Pain is a public health problem of substantial impact. It affects more than 100 million Americans each year—more than the total affected by heart disease, cancer, and diabetes combined—and is estimated to cost the Nation $560-$635 billion each year in medical costs and lost productivity.[2] While an important part of pain management, pharmaceutical approaches may provide incomplete relief and can carry serious side effects, including overmedication and opioid dependency and, in some cases, addiction. Commonly prescribed opioid pain relievers can be dangerous as even a single large dose can cause severe respiratory depression and death. Deaths from opioid pain relievers exceed those attributed to cocaine and heroin combined. Finding alternatives for pain management is needed.[3]

In 2011, after examining pain as a national public health problem, the Institute of Medicine (IOM) released a Consensus Report in 2011, entitled "Relieving Pain in America: A Blueprint for Transforming Prevention, Care, Education, and Research." The IOM report encourages Federal and state agencies and private organizations to accelerate the collection of data on pain incidence, prevalence, and treatments, and to take steps to develop integrative pain management strategies. The report notes that ideally, most patients with severe persistent pain would obtain care from an interdisciplinary team using an integrated approach that would target multiple dimensions of chronic pain—including disease management, reduction in pain severity, improved functioning, and emotional well-being and health-related quality of life.

[1] Nahin RL, Barnes PM, Stussman BA, et al. *Costs of complementary and alternative medicine (CAM) and frequency of visits to CAM practitioners: United States, 2007.* CDC National Health Statistics Report #18. 2009.

[2] IOM (Institute of Medicine). 2011. *Relieving Pain in America: A Blueprint for Transforming Prevention, Care, Education, and Research.* Washington, DC: The National Academies Press.

[3] *Drug Facts: Prescription and Over-the-Counter Medications,* National Institute on Drug Abuse, National Institutes of Health, May 2013. http://www.drugabuse.gov/publications/drugfacts/prescription-over-counter-medications, accessed April 28, 2014.

In addition, the Federal Government created an Interagency Pain Research Coordinating Committee (IPRCC) to enhance pain research efforts and promote collaboration across the government, to advance our fundamental understanding of pain, and to improve pain-related treatment strategies. Members include representatives of the Departments of Health and Human Services, Veterans Affairs (VA), and Defense (DOD), the scientific and medical communities, the public, and stakeholder groups. I serve as one of the NIH representatives. The IPRCC is developing a comprehensive population health level strategy for pain prevention, treatment, management, and research. One of the first efforts of the IPRCC was a thorough analysis of pain research across Federal agencies, resulting in the recently released "2011 IPRCC Federal Pain Research Portfolio Analysis Report"[4] which revealed many areas of shared research interests between and across Federal entities, but no notable redundancies.

NCCAM participates in the NIH Pain Consortium to enhance and increase the coordination of pain research across NIH. The Consortium's efforts include targeted initiatives such as the development of the first clinically-based data registry to help identify pain management interventions that are most effective for specific patient-types with chronic pain, led by the National Institute on Drug Abuse (NIDA), and the creation of standard research measures to assess chronic low back pain, which was spearheaded by NCCAM.

To improve pain education in health professional schools, the Pain Consortium established 12 Centers of Excellence in Pain Education to advance teaching and provide comprehensive curricula about the pathophysiology of pain, its assessment, diagnosis, management, and treatment. The curricula include the latest research results in complementary and integrative pain management, factors that contribute to both under- and over-prescribing of pain medications, and how pain manifests itself differently by gender, by age, and in diverse populations. In addition, NIDA, Medscape Education, and the White House Office of National Drug Control Policy developed two continuing medical education courses on practical guidance for physicians and other clinicians in screening pain patients for substance use disorder risk factors before prescribing, and in identifying when patients are abusing their medications. The courses use videos that model effective communication about sensitive issues, without losing sight of addressing the pain. To date, more than 80,000 health care professionals have completed these courses.

At NCCAM, an increasing proportion of our research budget is dedicated to studies examining promising non-pharmacological approaches for pain management, including mindfulness meditation, spinal manipulation, massage, acupuncture, and exercise forms, such as yoga and Tai chi. Some of these approaches are already being recommended by the American College of Physicians and the American Pain Society in their guidelines for the diagnosis and treatment of low back pain. NCCAM is interested in better understanding how these interventions work, for what type of pain conditions, and the optimal methods of practice and delivery. We also support Centers of Excellence for Research on Complementary and Alternative Medicine that bring a multifaceted interdisciplinary approach to research on pain. In addition, NCCAM recently established a new intramural research program that focuses entirely on pain using state-of-the-art neuroimaging and other advanced technologies to study the mechanisms of pain including the role of emotions and attention on the modulation of pain.

Last year, NCCAM joined NIDA, the National Institute on Alcohol Abuse and Alcoholism, and DOD in a joint initiative to conduct research on prevention and health promotion interventions to prevent alcohol and other drug abuse and associated physical and psychological health problems in Veterans and military personnel. NCCAM also issued a solicitation, along with NIDA and the VA, specifically focused on complementary and integrative approaches to managing pain and other symptoms such as posttraumatic stress, Traumatic Brain Injury, substance use disorders, anxiety, and sleep disturbances often experienced by Veterans and military personnel. The initiative requested research approaches to study (a) mind-body interventions such as mindfulness- or meditation-based stress reduction approaches, (b) yoga, (c) acupuncture, (d) art therapy, (e) massage, and (f) cognitive-behavioral interventions. Grant applications are currently under review, and we look forward to funding multiple studies later this year. Research findings from these initiatives are expected to lead to enhanced patient care and improved pain and symptom management through better integration of evidence-based complementary approaches.

---

[4] National Institutes of Health, National Institute of Neurological Disorders and Stroke, Office of Pain Policy. *2011 IPRCC Federal Pain Research Portfolio. Analysis Report.* Available at iprcc.nih.gov/news/CC_Pain_Portfolio_Analysis_Report.pdf. Accessed April 28, 2014.

At my direction, a special Working Group of the National Advisory Council on Complementary and Alternative Medicine was recently formed to explore ways to foster rigorous research that will inform the use and incorporation of complementary approaches in military and veteran populations and promote collaboration among the VA, DOD, and NCCAM. The Working Group, chaired by Lloyd Michener, M.D., of Duke University, includes current and former VA and DOD officials. The group is charged with defining a research agenda for mind/body interventions for pain and symptom management, including identifying the most promising therapies and the next steps for development of large clinical trials. Experts will present perspectives of patients, Veterans, military personnel, and clinicians to help shape the Working Group's recommendations.

In summary, NIH and NCCAM are committed to improving understanding and treatment of pain and related conditions for all Americans including military personnel and Veterans. We expect research results to provide information to the public and health care providers and policymakers. I appreciate the opportunity to appear before this Committee, and I look forward to answering any questions. Thank you.

RESPONSE TO POSTHEARING QUESTIONS SUBMITTED BY HON. BERNARD SANDERS TO JOSEPHINE BRIGGS, M.D., DIRECTOR, NATIONAL CENTER FOR COMPLEMENTARY AND ALTERNATIVE MEDICINE, NATIONAL INSTITUTES OF HEALTH

COMPLEMENTARY AND ALTERNATIVE MEDICINE (CAM)

Question 1. What can be done to increase long-term programmatic research to help better understand CAM therapies and their impact on servicemembers and veterans?

Response. As the Federal Government's lead agency for scientific research on complementary practices and integrative health interventions, the National Center for Complementary and Alternative Medicine (NCCAM) is committed to greater understanding of the usefulness and safety of complementary and integrative health practices and their role in improving health and health care. Since 2010, NCCAM has been working with the Departments of Defense (DOD) and Veterans Affairs (VA) to explore opportunities for partnerships and collaborations.

After participating in workshops on complementary interventions for pain management with DOD and Post Traumatic Stress Disorder with VA, NCCAM issued a Funding Opportunity Announcement (FOA) in 2012, to encourage collaborations with DOD and VA researchers and clinicians to study integrative approaches to pain and symptom management in military and Veteran populations. Under this initiative, seven collaborations were funded to study modalities such as massage, acupuncture and chiropractic for musculoskeletal pain and post-traumatic headache, as well as Tai Chi and mindfulness for treating stress disorders, anxiety, and depression. In 2013, NCCAM participated in a FOA with the National Institute on Drug Abuse (NIDA) and DOD, to promote research on interventions to prevent alcohol and other drug abuse and associated physical and psychological health problems in military personnel and Veterans. NCCAM funded two research projects under this FOA, both involving the study of innovative interventions for pain management and to reduce substance abuse.

Last year, NCCAM issued three FOAs, along with NIDA and VA, to encourage research on the non-pharmacological management of pain and co-morbid conditions in military personnel and Veterans. NCCAM has committed two million dollars in Fiscal Year 2014, and hopes to fund studies exploring a variety of complementary interventions for pain management, including combined interventions for treating pain and substance abuse, bright light treatment, mindfulness training, and the use of mobile neurofeedback applications for pain management.

To guide future collaborative efforts with DOD and VA, NCCAM recently established a special Working Group of the National Advisory Council on Complementary and Alternative Medicine. The Working Group is charged with advising NCCAM on potential collaborations, opportunities and strategies for integrative health research within DOD and VA health care settings. Invited experts will present perspectives of patients, military personnel and Veterans, clinicians, researchers, and policymakers to inform the Working Group in shaping its final recommendations. The Working Group is expected to submit a report to the National Advisory Council for Complementary and Alternative Medicine in early 2015.

NCCAM looks forward to building on current collaborations and continuing to partner with other NIH Institutes and Centers, DOD, and VA to further investigate the usefulness and safety of complementary and integrative health interventions for servicemembers and Veterans.

Question 2. A challenge of medical research is the length of time it takes for research to move from bench to bedside. What is the National Center for Complementary and Alternative Medicine doing specifically—and NIH more generally—to expedite this process?

Response. NCCAM is committed to improving the translation of research findings into improved public health. At NCCAM's core is a vision in which rigorous scientific evidence about complementary health practices informs both the decisions Americans make regarding the use of these health practices and their potential integration into health care. As such, NCCAM funds research across the continuum of basic, translational, efficacy, and effectiveness research. As part of our translational portfolio, NCCAM supports research required to design and implement definitive clinical research and "real-world" outcomes and effectiveness research that capitalizes on the reality that many complementary health interventions are in widespread public use. This research includes identifying and validating biomarkers or other signatures of biological effect; developing and validating measures of outcome; validating treatment algorithms and measures of quality control; and developing preliminary clinical evidence.

Additionally, NCCAM is leading the Health Care Systems Research Collaboratory, an NIH Common Fund initiative. This program is engaging health care delivery organizations as research partners, with the goal of strengthening the national capacity to conduct rigorous large-scale clinical trials in "real-world" settings. Through the Collaboratory, NIH is pioneering the development of approaches to conduct large-scale, cost-effective clinical research studies in the setting where patients already receive their care. Ultimately, this program could help increase the number and types of health care systems engaged in clinical research and enhance the relevance of research results to health care practice.

At the bedside-end of the continuum, NCCAM ensures that research results are widely disseminated to help the public make informed decisions about the use of complementary health practices and to enable health care providers to better manage patient care. NCCAM provides reliable, objective, and evidence-based information through a variety of approaches including emerging technology and platforms (i.e., video, social media, and mobile applications). Specifically for health care professionals, NCCAM's web site features a portal with links to scientific literature on complementary health practices, including reviews from the Cochrane Collaboration; clinical practice guidelines issued by third-party organizations; and online continuing education modules. In addition, NCCAM's monthly e-newsletter, NCCAM Clinical Digest, summarizes the state of the science on complementary health practices for specific health topics.

Across the NIH, many NIH Institutes and Centers and trans-NIH initiatives are also focused on expediting the process of turning observations in the laboratory and clinic into effective interventions that improve the health of the individual and the public—from diagnostics and therapeutics to medical procedures and behavioral changes. For example, the newest Center at NIH, the National Center for Advancing Translational Sciences (NCATS) was established to transform this process by catalyzing the generation of innovative methods and technologies that will enhance the development, testing, and implementation of diagnostics and therapeutics across a wide range of human diseases and conditions. Advances from NCATS are aimed at enabling researchers throughout the public and private sectors to more efficiently develop treatments for diseases, demonstrate effectiveness in improving health, and accelerate the pace at which new treatments are delivered to patients.

OPIOID USAGE

Question 3. How can collaborative efforts, such as the Interagency Pain Research Coordinating Committee, be leveraged to reduce the American health care system's dependency on high-dose medications to reduce chronic pain and mental health conditions?

Response. Collaborative efforts across the National Institutes of Health (NIH) and the Federal Government to increase the understanding of pain are helping to enable the development of novel therapies, including non-pharmacological approaches to treat those who suffer from pain conditions. Better strategies for the management of chronic pain may also reduce symptoms associated with some mental health conditions, such as depression and anxiety that are often comorbid with pain.

The Interagency Pain Research Coordinating Committee (IPRCC) was created to enhance pain research efforts and promote collaboration across the Federal Government, with the ultimate goal of advancing fundamental understanding of pain and improving pain-related treatment strategies.[1] The Committee comprises seven Federal members and 12 non-Federal members, six drawn from the scientific and medical communities and six from public and stakeholder groups. Six Federal Agencies are involved in this effort.[2] NCCAM is one of the NIH representatives.

The IPRCC conducted a thorough analysis of the Fiscal Year 2011 Federal pain research portfolio and released a report that identified areas for potential collaboration among the IPRCC- represented agencies. The analysis and accompanying report provide important tools to assist in sharing resources across the pain research community and for enhancing pain research efforts. For example, the Office of Pain Policy at NIH's National Institute on Neurological Disorders and Stroke, under the auspices of the IPRCC, launched the Federal Government's pain research database on May 27, 2014. This resource provides the public and the research community with an important tool to learn more about the breadth and details of pain research supported across the Federal Government.

The IPRCC is also charged with developing the National Pain Strategy, a comprehensive population health level strategy for pain prevention, treatment, management, and research. One objective of the strategy is to describe how efforts across Government agencies, including public-private partnerships, can be established, coordinated, and integrated to encourage population-focused research, education, communication, and community-wide approaches that can help reduce pain and its consequences. The development of the National Pain Strategy will involve coordination between the IPRCC and the NIH's Pain Consortium, as well as private-sector participants.

Within the NIH, the NIH Pain Consortium helps coordinate and support a number of pain research initiatives and activities across the NIH. Importantly, the Pain Consortium is cosponsoring a workshop with the NIH Office of Disease Prevention to address several issues related to pain management, including the long-term effectiveness of opioids for treating chronic pain and the use and effectiveness of opioid management strategies in minimizing opioid addiction, abuse, and misuse, maximizing pain relief, and improving patients' quality of life. Based on the evidence presented, an independent panel of experts will release a comprehensive report in early 2015 on the state of the evidence, identifying research gaps and proposing research priorities.

The efforts of the Pain Consortium have already made an impact. On May 21, 2014, NIH announced that the NIH Pain Consortium's first pain care curriculum—part of the 12 "Centers of Excellence in Pain Education"—showed significant improvements in medical student clinical skills.[3] The educational materials are designed to advance the assessment, diagnosis, and safe treatment of pain, while minimizing risks of abuse and addiction. The curricula include the latest research results in complementary and integrative pain management, factors that contribute to both under- and over-prescribing of pain medications, and how pain manifests itself differently by gender, by age, and in diverse populations. In addition, NIDA, Medscape Education, and the White House Office of National Drug Control Policy developed two continuing medical education courses on practical guidance for physicians and other clinicians in screening pain patients for substance use disorder risk factors before prescribing, and in identifying when patients are abusing their medications. The courses use videos that model effective communication about sensitive issues, without losing sight of addressing the pain. To date, more than 80,000 health care professionals have completed these courses. These efforts will help current and future health care professionals build clinical skills to better support, manage and treat patients with pain.

RESPONSE TO POSTHEARING QUESTIONS SUBMITTED BY HON. MARK BEGICH TO JOSEPHINE BRIGGS, M.D., DIRECTOR, NATIONAL CENTER FOR COMPLEMENTARY AND ALTERNATIVE MEDICINE, NATIONAL INSTITUTES OF HEALTH

Question 4. I know I hear from Veteran's in my state that ask for more alternative methods for pain, PTSD and with our large native population, many native veterans rely on native healers, in the Native Health Care system, they are called doctors. Have you researched the use of Native healing and if not will you be looking at this effective method of healing?

[1] http://www.iprcc.nih.gov
[2] DOD, VA, and within HHS, NIH, the Agency for Healthcare Research and Quality, the Centers for Disease Control and Prevention, and the Food and Drug Administration.
[3] http://www.nih.gov/news/health/may2014/nida-21.htm

43

Response. NCCAM is committed to studying the usefulness, safety and efficacy of complementary and integrative health approaches, many of which have origins in traditional healing practices. Although a wide variety of these practices are used by the American public, better information is needed on how or whether they work.

According to the Centers for Disease Control and Prevention, over 50 percent of American Indian/Alaska Native (AI/AN) adults use complementary therapies—greater than any other ethnic group.[4] Given the prevalence of complementary therapies among this population, research on native healing practices is important, and NCCAM takes a number of approaches to encourage such research. For example, NCCAM is interested in research projects utilizing systems of healing and health practices outside the conventional medical care and those studying the extent and use of self-care and integrative health practices, conventional medical care, or a combination of the two. Examples of NCCAM funded research projects include:

• "Drum-Assisted Recovery Therapy for Native Americans," Daniel Lee Dickerson, D.O., MPH, University of California, Los Angeles. Dr. Dickerson' grant focused on developing and pilot testing a treatment approach that included Drum Circles and the 12-steps of Alcoholics Anonymous within the conceptual framework of the Native American Medicine Wheel.

• "Chemopreventative Properties of Medicinal and Food Plants of the Lumbee Tribe," Tracie Locklear, Ph.D., University of Illinois, Chicago. Dr. Locklear's grant supported her research on the development and testing of natural agents isolated from medicinal and food plants of the Lumbee Tribe. The long term goal of the project was to develop new and novel natural agents for the chemoprevention of breast cancer.

In addition, NCCAM participates in the Native American Research Centers for Health (NARCH),[5] which is a partnership between the Indian Health Service and NIH. The goal of the NARCH program is to provide opportunities for tribes and tribal organizations to conduct research, research training, and faculty development that meet the needs of AI/AN communities.

[4] Barnes PM, Bloom B, Nahin R. CDC National Health Statistics Report #12. Complementary and Alternative Medicine Use Among Adults and Children: United States, 2007. December 2008.
[5] http://www.nigms.nih.gov/Training/NARCH/Pages/default.aspx

ADDITIONAL INFORMATION FROM JOSEPHINE P. BRIGGS, M.D., DIRECTOR, NATIONAL CENTER FOR COMPLEMENTARY AND ALTERNATIVE MEDICINE, PUBLIC HEALTH SERVICE, NATIONAL INSTITUTES OF HEALTH

 DEPARTMENT OF HEALTH & HUMAN SERVICES

Public Health Service
National Institutes of Health

National Center for Complementary
and Alternative Medicine
31 Center Drive
Building 31, Room 2B-11
Bethesda, Maryland 20892-2182
nccam.nih.gov

May 9, 2014

The Honorable Bernie Sanders
Chairman
Committee on Veterans' Affairs
412 Russell Senate Office Building
Washington, DC 20150

The Honorable Richard Burr
Ranking Member
Committee on Veterans' Affairs
825A Hart Senate Office Building
Washington, DC 20150

Dear Chairman Sanders and Ranking Member Burr:

Thank you for the opportunity to submit additional information for the record of the Senate Committee on Veterans' Affairs April 30, 2014 hearing "Overmedication: Problems and Solutions."

As I mentioned in my written testimony, the National Center for Complementary and Alternative Medicine (NCCAM), in partnership with the Department of Defense (DOD), Department of Veterans' Affairs (VA), the National Institute on Drug Abuse (NIDA), and the National Institute on Alcohol Abuse and Alcoholism (NIAAA), supports research on the use of complementary and integrative therapies for the management of pain and substance abuse in U.S. military personnel, Veterans, and their families. Our major initiatives to date include:

- Collaborative Activities to Promote Research on Integrative Approaches to Symptom Management in Military Populations, Administrative Supplement (PA-12-160);

- Prevention and Health Promotion Intervention to Prevent Alcohol and Other Drug Abuse and Associated Physical and Psychological Health Problems in U.S. Military Personnel, Veterans and their Families (RFA-DA-13-013); and

- Studies of Non-pharmacological Approaches to Managing Pain and Co-Morbid Conditions in U.S. Military Personnel, Veterans, and their Families (RFA-AT-14-003; RFA-AT-14-004; RFA-AT-005).

Attached is additional information about the grants awarded under the first two initiatives. We look forward to funding grants under the third, later this year. Please let me know if you have any questions or would like additional information.

Sincerely,

Josephine P. Briggs, M.D.
Director

Attachments

- **Collaborative Activities to Promote Research on Integrative Approaches to Symptom Management in Military Populations,** Administrative Supplement (PA-12-160) http://grants.nih.gov/grants/guide/pa-files/PA-12-160.html. Sponsor: NCCAM only. NCCAM funded seven supplements to ongoing NCCAM-funded grants (parent grants).

  1. Title: "Central Mechanisms of Body Based Intervention for Musculoskeletal Low Back Pain"
     Principal Investigator: Mark Bishop, Ph.D.
     Institution: University of Florida, Gainesville
     Grant #: 5R01AT006334-02S1
     Parent grant: Examine the mechanisms of spinal manipulation and body-based interventions for low back pain using state-of-the-art techniques for examining pain sensitivity, such as quantitative sensory testing and functional magnetic resonance imaging of the brain.
     Supplement: Expand pilot study to include Veterans.

  2. Title: "Integrative Care for Chronic Musculoskeletal Pain in VA Hospitals and Clinics"
     Principal Investigator: Lynn Debar, Ph.D., M.P.H.
     Institution: Kaiser Foundation Research Institution, Oakland, California
     Grant #: R01AT005896-02S1
     Parent grant: Evaluate use of acupuncture and chiropractic care for the treatment of chronic pain within an integrated health plan.
     Supplement: Assess the feasibility of identifying delivery of complementary and integrative health approaches to Veterans with musculoskeletal disorder.

  3. Title: "Effect of Complementary and Alternative Medicine on Pain Among Inpatients"
     Principal Investigator: Jeffery Dusek, Ph.D.
     Institution: Allina Health System, Minneapolis, Minnesota
     Grant #: R01AT006518-02S1
     Parent grant: Evaluate the effectiveness of complementary and integrative health therapies for pain management in an acute care inpatient hospital.
     Supplement: Develop a new collaboration to assess feasibility of expanding complementary and integrative health services at the Ann Arbor VA.

  4. Title: "Multisite RCT Investigating the Efficacy of Massage in Osteoarthritis"
     Principal Investigator: Adam Perlman, M.D., M.P.H.
     Institution: Duke University, Durham, North Carolina
     Grant #: 5R01AT004623-05S2
     Parent grant: Randomized controlled trial to assess the duration of therapeutic effect of eight weeks of Swedish massage and maintenance dosing for treatment of knee pain in subjects with osteoarthritis.
     Supplement: Expand study to include 25 Veterans.

  5. Title: "Neuroimaging Biomarkers of Mind-Body Treatment in Post-Traumatic Headache"
     Principal Investigators: Kirsten Tillisch, M.D., Bruce Naliboff, Ph.D.
     Institution: University of California, Los Angeles
     Grant #: R01AT007137-02S1

<u>Parent grant:</u> Seek to validate biomarkers using brain imaging to serve as objective, reliable measures to identify response to mindfulness based stress reduction and assess symptom improvement in chronic visceral pain.
<u>Supplement:</u> Using MBSR and imaging, develop protocols for recruitment and screening of Veterans with post-traumatic headache.

6. Title: "Tai Chi Mind Body Exercise in Treatment of Post-Traumatic Stress Disorder"
   Principal Investigator: Chenchen Wang, M.D.
   Institution: Tufts Medical Center, Boston, Massachusetts
   Grant #: R01AT006367-02S2
   <u>Parent:</u> Evaluate benefits of Tai Chi for fibromyalgia in comparison to standard exercise therapy.
   <u>Supplement:</u> Establish a protocol for Tai Chi for post-traumatic stress disorder, develop relationships with collaborators, research literature, and conduct focus groups.

7. Title: "Mindfulness Based Stress Reduction and Cognitive Function in Stress and Aging"
   Principal Investigator: Julie Wetherell, Ph.D.
   Institution: University of California at San Diego
   Grant #: R34AT007070-02S1
   <u>Parent grant:</u> Evaluate the feasibility of adapting and testing mindfulness based stress reduction for improving clinical outcomes and cognitive function in older adults with anxiety disorders or depression.
   <u>Supplement:</u> Expand study to include Veterans with anxiety disorders, depression, or traumatic brain injury.

- **Prevention and Health Promotion Intervention to Prevent Alcohol and Other Drug Abuse and Associated Physical and Psychological Health Problems in U.S. Military Personnel, Veterans and their Families.** (R34 RFA-DA-13-013) http://grants.nih.gov/grants/guide/rfa-files/RFA-DA-13-013.html. Cosponsors: NIDA, NIAAA, NCCAM, and DOD's Office of the Assistant Secretary for Health Affairs. NCCAM is funding two grants:

  1. Title: "Screening, Brief Intervention, and Referral to Treatment for Pain Management (SBIRT-PM) for Veterans Filing Compensation Claims"
     Principal Investigator: Marc I. Rosen, M.D.
     Institution: Yale University, New Haven, Connecticut
     Grant #: R34AT-008318-01
     Summary: Many Veterans return from military service with painful injuries and apply for disability compensation. These Veterans are often at risk for substance abuse disorders. This grant will fund a clinical study examining whether a counseling intervention administered to Veterans with musculoskeletal pain at their Compensation and Pension evaluation examination impacts their substance use.

  2. Title: "Improving Opioid Safety in Veterans Using Collaborative Care and Decision Support"
     Principal Investigator: Karen H. Seal, M.D., M.P.H.
     Institution: Northern California Institute for Research and Education, San Francisco, California
     Grant #: R34AT008319
     Summary: Most opioid are prescribed in primary care where many chronic pain patients, including Veterans, also present with substance abuse and other mental health problems. These additional issues put them at high risk for adverse clinical outcomes, such as opioid overdose. This grant will support the development and preliminary testing of a collaborative care intervention that may improve safety in opioid prescribing and pain management. In the intervention, the care manager will assist primary care providers by using motivational interviewing to communicate decision support guidelines to Veterans with chronic pain.

48

- **Studies of Non-pharmacological Approaches to Managing Pain and Co-Morbid Conditions in U.S. Military Personnel, Veterans, and their Families.** Cosponsors: NCCAM, NIDA, and VA's Health Services Research & Development Service (HSR&D). NCCAM expects to fund three or four grants, and is committed to spending two million dollars in Fiscal Year 2014. NIDA and VA also may fund several grants.

1. **Clinical Trials and Interventional Studies. (R01) RFA-AT-14-003.**
   http://grants.nih.gov/grants/guide/rfa-files/RFA-AT-14-003.html.
   NCCAM and NIDA issued this Funding Opportunity Announcement (FOA) to accelerate clinical trial or interventional research on non-pharmacological approaches to symptom management for pain and associated problems among U.S. military personnel, Veterans, and their families.

2. **Pilot and Feasibility Studies. (R34) RFA-AT-14-004.**
   http://grants.nih.gov/grants/guide/rfa-files/RFA-AT-14-004.html.
   This FOA, issued by NCCAM and NIDA, will support preliminary clinical studies needed for planning and design of subsequent studies or clinical efficacy/effectiveness trials.

3. **Health Services and Observational Studies. (R01) RFA-AT-14-005.**
   http://grants.nih.gov/grants/guide/rfa-files/RFA-AT-14-005.html.
   This FOA was issued by NCCAM, NIDA and VA's HSR&D to accelerate health services and observational research on non-pharmacological approaches to symptom management for pain and associated problems among U.S. military personnel and Veterans.

Chairman SANDERS. Dr. Briggs, thank you very much.

Let me begin with Dr. Petzel. Dr. Briggs, I think appropriately, talked about this issue as an epidemic. We have a horrific problem in Vermont but I think it is shared in States throughout this country. People overdosing, getting addicted, turning to crime, self-destruction. It is an awful issue.

As we know, as bad as this problem is for the civilian population, it is likely even worse among our military and veteran population, largely because of the nature of the injuries and conditions they experience.

Dr. Petzel, first, how serious is the problem you are addressing and second—Dr. Gaudet and maybe Dr. Marshall might want to join in—tell me the role that you think complementary and alternative medicine can play in addressing those problems.

Dr. PETZEL. Thank you, Mr. Chairman.

First of all, in terms of the magnitude of the problem, several have mentioned it. We estimate that 50 percent of veterans that are coming to us seeking care have some sort of pain. Much of it is musculoskeletal, back injuries, et cetera, associated with the work that a soldier, sailor, airman, and Marine may be doing.

We are prescribing opioids for somewhere around 650,000 veterans at the present time which is a large number of people, and we recognize the fact that this is an issue that has to be addressed very directly.

I would like to just take a minute before I turn to the other panel members to describe the opioid safety program that we are involved in to try and get a grip on and reduce the use of opiates which, by the way, has reduced the number of patients receiving opioids in the last 18 months by 50,000. Still, there are a lot of people getting it but——

Chairman SANDERS. So, 50,000 fewer veterans are now receiving opioids?

Dr. PETZEL. That is correct.

The five things that are the central part of the pain management program are: one, every medical center has to have a pain management clinic; two, every medical center has a pain consultation service. VA requires the use of integrative CAM approaches.

The details of this—we require the use of the step care model which was developed in the VA and I think has been adopted by the Department of Defense now which begins with, in the primary care clinic, self-management and management in primary care of pain. If needed, it moves to the secondary pain clinic; and then finally, there are tertiary pain services available.

The centerpiece of this, though, is the opioid dashboard, monthly report to the facilities, to the providers in the facility, and to the pain management point of contact about people that are prescribing outside of the standard and patients that are taking medication outside of the standard.

That is followed by education and discussion and consultation with the providers to bring their use of opioids into the standard.

Chairman SANDERS. OK. If I can interrupt you, we will take a little bit more time for everybody, because we only have four of us here. But I wonder—if it is OK with you, Dr. Petzel, I wanted to shift over to Dr. Gaudet and Dr. Marshall.

What are you doing with complementary and alternative medicine and is it, in fact, working?

Dr. GAUDET. Thank you, Chairman Sanders.

I think you are aware that the vision for health care, as Ranking Member Burr referenced, is personalized proactive patient-driven; central to that are strategies that are inclusive of complementary approaches that empower the veteran to take into their own hands whether they have pain issues. Of course, this expands far beyond pain to the many, many conditions facing veterans and the public, complex conditions where a simple fix does not exist.

So, I think that these areas, particularly pain, are phenomenal places where the VA is committed to bringing more holistic approaches to veterans. The veterans are finding them very empowering, very much an asset to the complement of what they can do to address their issues of pain as well as other issues. Yes sir.

Chairman SANDERS. In English.

Dr. GAUDET. Yes, sorry.

Chairman SANDERS. What are you offering the patient? So, somebody walks in. They have chronic pain. They are concerned about overmedication. You are concerned. What therapies are you offering and are they, in fact, working?

These are fairly radical ideas in a certain sense, yes? Or not?

Dr. GAUDET. I do not know how radical they are, but I think that the therapies that are most promising and most often utilized right now in the VA are very parallel to the DOD and the public.

So, they tend to be mind-body approaches such as meditation, acupuncture, movement therapies such as, yoga, tai chi, spinal manipulation. These are the general approaches that seem to have the greatest promise—relatively noninvasive and at low risk.

Chairman SANDERS. Now, I have been impressed. I have been to VA facilities all over the country and I have been to a couple of DOD facilities and I am amazed. You know, 20 or 30 years ago I think it is fair to say that if we were talking about this list of therapies, people would have thought there were a few folks in California or certain other places utilizing them, not the U.S. Department of Defense or VA.

So, in terms of treatments like acupuncture, are they working? What can you tell us about your success rates? Does it work?

Dr. GAUDET. I think the most evidence actually exists for acupuncture as it relates to pain. Our research office of evidence-based synthesis just finished a comprehensive look at all the evidence related to acupuncture. It is a very useful document because it basically says where is there evidence for the use of acupuncture, do we know, and is it of benefit or do we know it is not of benefit or there is a category where we just do not know yet, we do not have research.

The areas where there is the best and strongest evidence for acupuncture are pain, chronic pain, headaches, and migraines. So, it is a rational place to start.

Chairman SANDERS. All right. Dr. Marshall, if I walk into your beautiful facility in Minneapolis, and I was just there a few days ago, and I am in pain, what are my options other than drugs?

Dr. MARSHALL. Mr. Chairman, thank you for that question.

I would say at Minneapolis we view pain management as a full-spectrum opportunity to engage with a patient and move them toward a healthier and more functional life.

So, we have deployed various complementary and alternative modalities at different levels of our facility. For instance, nurses, we trained 900 nurses in January of this year; a 4-hour training in complementary and alternative medicine with integrative nursing.

Modalities that we trained specifically to those nurses included acupuncture, relaxation breathing, meditation, and essential oils or aroma therapy.

Chairman SANDERS. When you tell your patients these therapies are available, do they say, hey, I would like to try that? What do they say?

Dr. MARSHALL. There is a lot of variability. Some patients, you know, express a strong desire for opioid pain medications. Many patients, though, are very open once they learn that these alternatives are a standard part of our medical treatment armamentarium at Minneapolis VA. I think many patients are gravitating toward these kind of services.

Chairman SANDERS. Can you tell us some success stories? Are there people who have lived with pain, who were heavily medicated but because of complementary and alternative medicine have been able to get rid of medication? Dr. Marshall, do you have stories?

Dr. MARSHALL. Yes, I would like to talk briefly about a program that we have just started. This is part of the VA's efforts to have Council for Accreditation of Rehabilitation Facilities, CARF, pain rehab center at each VISN. So, we started one in January of this year.

We recruited the Director of the Mayo Clinic Pain Rehab Program who is now leading our efforts. So that program which is just starting at Minneapolis VA had seven veterans, four of them were on opioids, three of them were tapered off, and one was tapered down.

And a cornerstone of that program is a 3-week intensive residential program and a cornerstone of that program is activating patients' innate healing abilities through use of primarily complementary and alternative modalities, including cognitive behavioral therapy, meditation, relaxation breathing, tai chi, yoga, and other active forms.

Chairman SANDERS. So, you have some specific indications that these therapies are working?

Dr. MARSHALL. Yes.

Chairman SANDERS. OK. I have exceeded my time.

Senator Burr.

Senator BURR. Thank you, Mr. Chairman.

Dr. Petzel, just one follow-up to this hope that we get a pathway on Phoenix to some facts. When we had one death at the Columbia VA medical center that was related to delays, when the medical center and the VISN leadership became aware of that problem there were four outside reviews, specifically the task force, the Office of Medical Inspector, and the IG.

Are you confident that we have the sufficient focus on Phoenix for this Committee and for the VA to understand what, if anything, went wrong?

Dr. PETZEL. Senator, I am. I think that the IG's presence, the inspector general, with their independent look, and they have a huge collection of manpower that they are focusing.

Senator BURR. What would trigger so many components for Columbia on one death versus just the IG on this?

Dr. PETZEL. I really cannot answer that. I do not know. We sent our team in. I think the IG actually went in twice. I really cannot speak specifically to what they did. But I am confident that the IG has the resources and has them present in Phoenix to get to the bottom of what has occurred there.

Senator BURR. OK. Dr. Gaudet, let me ask you. Is it easier to write a prescription or to try a CAM approach?

Dr. GAUDET. It is easier to write a prescription.

52

Senator BURR. Yes. Can you envision, any of you from the VA, that it would be appropriate to prescribe an opiate to somebody who, in their medical records, has an opiate addiction?

Dr. GAUDET. I am probably not the best person to answer that, not being a pain doctor.

Senator BURR. Dr. Marshall?

Dr. MARSHALL. I think the indications would be extremely rare. It would be very unusual to do that, but it might be done in certain situations, especially situations around acute pain from trauma after an operation.

Senator BURR. So, for a veteran with an opiate addiction being treated by VA and sent home for the weekend with 19 prescriptions, including 12 tablets of oxycodone, and 3 hours later he dies of a drug overdose; that would be an unusual circumstance?

Dr. MARSHALL. I would concur with your previous statement that one death too many. It should not happen.

Senator BURR. Dr. Petzel, VA issued a pain management directive in 2009 and in a House Veterans' Affairs Committee hearing last fall on the issue, Dr. Jesse said that all VISNs and VA facilities have implemented a pain management directive. Yet data obtained by the Center for Investigative Reporting shows, ''VA doctors are prescribing more opiates than ever and the data suggests adoption of the directive varies widely.''

This is not the only time we have heard problems about regulations and programs being executed inconsistently across the VA. What oversight does the VA central office perform to make sure that the new programs and directives issued are implemented as intended?

Dr. PETZEL. Thank you, Senator Burr.

One, the opioids safety initiative is intended to standardize the way we approach. Two, we have demonstrated that opioid prescribing in the VA has actually decreased, as I mentioned earlier, by 50,000 in the last approximately 18 months; and we expect to see that plummet. Number 3——

Senator BURR. We put this management plan into effect in 2009 and we had an upward spike. You will agree to that?

Dr. PETZEL. Yes.

If I could digress for a minute. In this country in general, not just the VA, there was 10–15 years ago a feeling that pain was not being adequately managed, and an effort was made to educate doctors about using opioids and other things to adequately manage pain, and I think in this country there was an overreaction to that phenomenon. And that is part of why we are involved in this effort to try and get a grip on opioid prescribing and to aggressively pursue other approaches to managing pain. While I was not here at the time, my suspicion is that that was part of what was going on within the VA.

Senator BURR. Well, I think Dr. Gaudet reinforced, I think, our belief, and I think it is the fact that it is easier to write a prescription than it is to go through a CAM process; and I think Dr. Briggs would probably agree with me.

There are some medical conditions that we probably will not be able to use an alternative for. The pain is real. It is consistent. It can only be addressed with some type of opiate medication or alternative to an opiate. For those people, they usually fall into a category of a specific illness that they have. Certainly, we do have some servicemembers that fall into that category.

Here is my concern, Dr. Petzel, and my question is this, when people do not follow the guidelines set by VA—be it a doctor, nurse, whoever—what tools do you have to hold them accountable?

I mean, we have seen difficulty with sterilization of medical devices. You and I have seen where insulin injection pens—multi-use injection pens—that we have now made a determination that we are not going to use them at the VA anymore because we——

Dr. PETZEL. No, they are not used in-patient. They are very, very deeply used as outpatients. They are great.

Senator BURR. Why do we not use them in-patient?

Dr. PETZEL. Because of the possibility that there might be confusion, as we talked about.

Senator BURR. Because we cannot with certainty believe that it is being executed by those guidelines, which means you cannot stick a different person with the same pen.

So, if something that simple is tough to do, what gives us confidence that we can carry out a pain management directive successfully or any other directive within the health care system?

Dr. PETZEL. Senator Burr, I would point out that the opioid dashboard is our tool for monitoring the prescriber's use of opioids. And the first step when somebody is not using these appropriately is to educate them about the way that it ought to be done properly.

So, do we have the tools to correct behavior that we think needs to be modified? Absolutely yes.

Senator BURR. OK, Mr. Chairman. Thank you.

Chairman SANDERS. Thank you.

Senator Begich.

**STATEMENT OF HON. MARK BEGICH,
U.S. SENATOR FROM ALASKA**

Senator BEGICH. Mr. Chairman, thank you very much. I know earlier you talked about the issue in Arizona so I just want to know that—assuming that as soon as the IG report comes, and I know, Mr. Chairman, you noted that we will have some sort of process here. Obviously, we will look forward to that.

The question that I am going to be very interested in, and it can be answered now or later, and that is the issue of the information that the Arizona VA was sending to the national, whatever the information was on appointment status; in other words, how long it took people to come through their appointments—that information. Was that correct or were there issues with it. That is going to be my question.

There are a lot of details of deaths and so forth. What I want to know is did the information that came from the VA in Arizona to the national—who keeps track of successes at the different VAs and the amount of backlog and appointment scheduling—on those metrics, will that report or other reports confirm accuracy in the delivery of that information. That is going to be my fundamental question.

Dr. PETZEL. Senator Begich, as I mentioned earlier, we had a team down there looking in a preliminary fashion at the cir-

54

cumstances in Phoenix, and to date we have not found that there is any discrepancy between the information that we were aware of and were getting and the information as it actually existed in Phoenix.

We have found no evidence for a secret list and we have not found any evidence to-date that anybody died while sitting on the waiting list.

Senator BEGICH. Understood. And the IG is looking at all those questions I am assuming?

Dr. PETZEL. Yes, they are; as near as I know, yes.

Senator BEGICH. OK. And I apologize. I know this part was answered. What is their timetable? Do you know?

Dr. PETZEL. They have not shared that with us, so I do not know.

Senator BEGICH. OK. We will probably hear details as time moves on.

Dr. PETZEL. I hope.

Senator BEGICH. OK. Thank you. I missed one meeting—I cannot remember if I was here or at the Appropriations Committee—but I wanted again to commend you all for working on and reviewing the NUKA model in Alaska.

We think this is—as we talk about overmedication and many other things—I think they have really capitalized on a very unique model that is looking at the whole body and all people engaged in health care. One of the things that I want to ask is, I am assuming in this issue today that we are talking about, overmedication, as you look at the NUKA model you will be also looking at this piece of the equation.

For example, I know they use not only alternative medicines but they also use through the native health care, native healing methods. Is that also something as you look at the NUKA model you can be examining because I want to make sure that is part of the equation.

Dr. PETZEL. My understanding, Senator Begich, is the central feature of the NUKA model is listening to the patient's story and then crafting the therapy around that individual patient's story and their circumstance. Since it is an Alaskan native program, those medicines, et cetera, are woven intimately into the way they deliver care.

In the Native community here in the States where the VA is dealing, we also employ native healers, et cetera, and those concepts in dealing with that particular patient population. But I think Dr. Gaudet can maybe comment briefly on the fact that that is a tone that goes through our program.

Dr. GAUDET. Yes, thank you, Senator. I would certainly just underscore the importance of this holistic approach which I appreciate your question actually brings to the surface.

I think the challenge before us really—truly not just in VA health care but nationally in the model of health care that is dominant in this country—it is so much easier to write a prescription, as Ranking Member Burr said.

The system is designed to do that. We as physicians are trained to find it-fix it. I can operate and I can write you a prescription and anything outside of that—and this is a slight exaggeration—but I am not actually trained to think about or understand.

So, this transformation is a huge system change, and it does as you have described and as Dr. Petzel has described, begin with understanding the person. If we are in a situation such as Senator Boozman, thank goodness we have the high-tech approach. Perfect. They can go in. We can sew you up. We can fix the problem.

Senator BEGICH. Right.

Dr. GAUDET. But in the myriad of things like pain, like obesity, like PTSD, those find it-fix it cures do not exist. So, this holistic approach starting with the individual, understanding their cultural beliefs and creating a personalized approach for and with them is absolutely essential.

Senator BEGICH. Very good. Let me proceed, if I can, because I have limited time here. General, I know the Army and TRICARE have recently required mental health counselors to our veterans be credited through the Council for Accreditation of Counseling Related Educational Programs.

Here is the challenge in Alaska. We do not have the capacity to meet those standards because of the uniqueness of Alaska. It is not offered in Alaska, so it makes it difficult; and with huge gaps in mental health professional numbers, how can we go with this when in reality we have vacancies that we should fill which can easily be filled with qualified counselors. But how are we going to meet this in Alaska?

I mean, I know everyone likes a one-size-fits-all solution. Those do not work in Alaska. I will tell you there is no better health care as what the VA is looking—Indian Health Services—no better health care delivery system in the country. So, we figured out how to do it and it does not come from a national model. It does not come from the standards that people sit around and make up.

I mean, we deal with reality. That is why we have a great dental program in the Indian Health Services. You know, the dental community does not necessarily like it totally, nationally, but it works in Alaska because we have remote areas and we have huge tooth decay and other things that we have been able to accomplish through dental therapists.

So, how are we going to handle this?

Chairman SANDERS. In 24 seconds.

General COOTS. Yes, sir. Alaska is known for its use of tele-medicine initiatives, and I think that for the military utilizing tele-behavioral health is probably one of the biggest initiatives that we have in serving areas that are remote or where we do not have those health care providers.

We are looking at some different ways of attracting additional behavioral health providers. We are also looking at training some of our own. As we draw down the military, we have a large core of physicians assistants that we are looking at retrainings some of them as behavioral health physicians' assistants.

Senator BEGICH. Very good. Let me say, Mr. Chairman, I have a couple of cases which I am going to send to Dr. Petzel and maybe some very specific questions on how we would respond to these kind of individuals that deal with medication.

Thank you very much.

Chairman SANDERS. Thank you, Senator Begich.

Senator Isakson.

Senator ISAKSON. General Coots, first of all, thank you for your service particularly at Walter Reed. You all performed miracles on a daily basis in rehab for our servicemen. We appreciate it very much.

I know Colonel Galloway's responsibilities are rehabilitation and reintegration of DOD active duty troops back into society I take it or back into the military?

General COOTS. Both.

Senator ISAKSON. Which tells me that opiate overprescription is probably as big a problem in DOD as it is in veterans' health care. Is that correct?

General COOTS. Sir, I would say we have statistics that show that up until about 2011, about 26 percent of all active duty were on some level of opioid medications, either one single opioid or multiple opioids.

The Army is traditionally a little bit higher, 2 or 3 percentage points higher, I think, by the nature of what we do and the pain that our servicemembers have from repeated combat tours in remote areas.

But all the statistics are showing now that with a big push for cultural change, with integration of these alternative medical modalities, that we are seeing a downturn in opioid use across the military, particularly across the Army, and then a large upswing from 10 percent up to 28 percent now, utilizing alternative medicine.

Senator ISAKSON. Which is my point because, you know, we use DOD for all kinds of medical research: breast cancer, prostate cancer, things like that because you have a controlled environment. You have people who are not necessarily voluntarily participating but they are participating because it is their job. We get a lot of medical data.

I guess we have learned from addiction and opioid overuse that the "settled science" is there in terms of what constitutes an addiction or an overuse. What we are trying to do is find out how we deal with it, and once it happens, to prevent it from happening again. Is that right?

General COOTS. Yes, Senator, that is correct.

Senator ISAKSON. Then that brings me to my question. Seamless transition from DOD health care to veterans health care, which by the way General Schoomaker did a remarkable job of improving in his service at Walter Reed and in the military.

What is DOD doing as these active duty military personnel go into veteran status? What is the transition like particularly with regard to opiates and then opiates having been prescribed, of them having been addicted? Is there a program or do they go into a black hole and the VA just has to discover the problem all for themselves?

General COOTS. Senator, that is a good question. I will answer it in two parts.

First, we have a shared formulary where we have lined up the formulary so that any medications that a military member might be on, as they transition into the veterans health care system, that same medication or modality is available to them in the transition.

We also are working on improving our warm handoff such that our military servicemembers have a lead coordinator. There is a corresponding lead coordinator on the VA side so that their information is transmitted directly in a handoff from that military lead coordinator to the VA system so that all of the associated and ancillary modalities that have treated them for whatever their problems are, be it opiate, be it anything else, all of those will transfer over so there is a knowledge transfer.

So, there is no falling off in the cracks or going into a black hole.

Senator ISAKSON. Good. Good.

Dr. Marshall, the opioid safety initiative started in Minneapolis, is that right?

Dr. MARSHALL. That is correct, Senator.

Senator ISAKSON. If you uncover a provider who is not following the proper safety administration of opioid prescriptions, what training or what follow-up do you require to make sure that they do not do it again, or is there a prescription for doing that?

Dr. MARSHALL. Well, first of all, Senator, thank you for that question because I think it is an integral part of what is happening at Minneapolis. So, we are building a standard of care and a cultural change in how we prescribe opioids.

Part of it is building the prescribing of opioids into a team setting so we are using the providers who are doing the prescribing, the pharmacists who bring their unique skill set to the primary care team to help monitor for adverse effects or, you know, dosage problems, and also mental health. So, a lot of the control happens at that point working with the patient and the primary care team.

Another phase of the accountability process is that we have transparent data—the dashboard that Dr. Petzel mentioned. So, we are using that to understand who are the outlying prescribers who need more help with changing their prescribing patterns.

And the final stage of accountability rests with the chief of staff who, at our facility, has been very involved in providing specific direction to providers who are outside of the standard of care.

So, it is a supportive system but there are levels of accountability.

Senator ISAKSON. Dr. Petzel, you are familiar with our question with regard to suicide in the Atlanta VA, and I appreciate very much your attention to the ongoing initiative there.

But it occurred to me that in the Atlanta VA situation where there were four instances now taking place over the last year, two of those were non-drug addicted Vietnam-era, noncombat veterans, meaning that they were veterans who served during the Vietnam era—my age group, in their late 60s or early 70s. They were not in combat. They did not transition from DOD to VA health care recently. They did it over a long period of time.

I worry sometimes that prescribing opiates to mental health patients who come in for their first encounters at VA prescribing opiates might mask a greater problem or might accelerate a problem that exists.

Is there any disciplinary requirements within the VA as far as mental health encounters are concerned in terms of prescribing opiates?

58

Dr. PETZEL. Senator Isakson, that is an excellent question. There are certain antecedents that are frequently found in patients who have either attempted suicide or actually committed suicide. Depression, PTSD, sleep disorders, and pain. Pain is often an antecedent to suicide, particularly chronic pain.

So, the mental health provider is attuned to the fact that when they see somebody who is new to them that they need to be evaluated for those antecedents to be sure that they are taken into account when they begin to write prescriptions.

So, anybody who has mental health problems who then also presents with a pain problem requires and gets very special attention.

Senator ISAKSON. Thank you.

Thank you, Mr. Chairman.

Chairman SANDERS. Thank you, Senator Isakson.

Senator Blumenthal.

Senator BLUMENTHAL. General Coots, you mentioned a statistic before which I missed as to the percentage of use of opioids. I think that was the percentage in the Army or the military. Could you repeat that?

General COOTS. Yes, Senator. Up to 2011, the number was about 26 percent of all active duty had been prescribed at least one opioid medication.

Senator BLUMENTHAL. And that could be in the course of the individual soldier's entire service? Or over what period of time?

General COOTS. We are actually tracking that on a year by year basis, watching it; and over time, say, from 2007 to 2011, you saw a steady increase up to that 26 percent point. After about 2011 over the last 2 years, going on almost 3 years, we have seen a steady drop off, either stabilization or decline in the numbers that are using it.

Senator BLUMENTHAL. So, let us take 2013. Over 2013, what percentage of active duty Army soldiers were prescribe some form of opioid?

General COOTS. Senator, I do not have that exact number.

Senator BLUMENTHAL. What is the last year for which you have a number?

General COOTS. Sir, actually I do. It looks like about 24 percent or so, about 24 percent in 2013. So, down from 26 percent in 2011.

Senator BLUMENTHAL. 26 percent in 2011 to 2013, 24 percent?

General COOTS. Yes, Senator.

Senator BLUMENTHAL. So, it is a pretty small difference.

General COOTS. It is a small difference but I think it still represents a big cultural change and a move ahead because over the war years you saw a steady increase in it and the war is not yet over. We are still getting casualties although fewer; but over those last few years, we have been able to use these alternative modalities to include battlefield acupuncture. We use intranasal ketamine on the battlefield now which decreases the amount of morphine that you have to use.

So, I think all of that is contributing as well in those complex casualties, and then translate that to our primary care clinics and our interdisciplinary pain management centers where we are implementing these alternative medications. I think all of that has been contributing to it.

So, we are right at the beginning of this cultural shift and this cultural change.

Senator BLUMENTHAL. Let me just make sure that I understand that number. That is total active duty soldiers.

General COOTS. That is total active duty.

Senator BLUMENTHAL. 26 percent were prescribed some form of opioid in 2011 and 24 percent in 2013. That is not injured soldiers. It is all soldiers.

General COOTS. That is all soldiers. This is all soldiers sailors, airmen, and Marines. That is all DOD.

Senator BLUMENTHAL. OK. Let me ask you. You mentioned the warm handoff from active duty service to separation and VA treatment. As you probably know, many of us on this Committee have been concerned about the lack of interoperability of the Army medical records with the VA records in terms of the electronic medical record systems that each has.

Do you see an effect of the lack of complete compatibility? I do not know what exactly the technical term would be, but I know that everybody is talking about trying to make it work better but still do not have an interoperable system.

Do you see an effect of that?

General COOTS. Actually, no, Senator. We are very compatible and very interoperable when it goes to that. There may be narrow pipelines between the two electronic health records but it still allows us to transition and transfer that critical information on complex patients and patients on——

Senator BLUMENTHAL. Is there an automatic re-evaluation when a soldier or an airman or Marine, or sailor goes from active duty to veteran status; re-evaluation of the prescription opioids?

In other words, does somebody say, well, you have been getting this medication or that, let us have a look here. Maybe we need to do something different.

General COOTS. To my understanding, there is an intake. Anytime you do a handoff or handover of a servicemember's care into the veterans' system, there is going to be an intake process.

We transition all of that information from that one lead coordinator to the next. But certainly when they get in and they have a new provider, a new team who is taking over, there is a re-evaluation of everything that has happened in that servicemember's medical history now than they have become a veteran.

That does not necessarily mean there is a change in therapeutic approach or a change in modalities but it certainly could mean that.

Senator BLUMENTHAL. It could mean it for an individual case.

Let me ask Secretary Petzel whether he has any observations.

Dr. PETZEL. Thank you, Senator Blumenthal.

A comment on a couple of things. First of all, we have ready access to everything that is electronic in the DOD records. The interoperability part, we are working toward being sure that things mean the same in each kind of record. So, that is improving. It is definitely improving.

Also the transition is improving with TAP, the Transition Assistance Program. We present to each one of the exiting servicemembers about what is available in DOD. People are often identified now in that program that need to have a warm handoff. We are seeing much more of the at-risk patients being handed off to VA in a warm fashion.

Senator BLUMENTHAL. Just so I understand, I use the term but what does that mean?

Dr. PETZEL. That means there is a specific call to a VA medical center, this patient, John Jones, is transiting into the VA health care system. This is who he is. Here is what it means. We need an appointment for him. That is a warm handoff.

What happens when they come to the VA—not all of them do, by the way. We need to understand that unfortunately we do not see as many people as we would like to see. They are evaluated. Our perspective as an organization is that we want to use the least risky, effective way of managing a patient's pain.

So that my hope would be and the expectation would be that their pain is evaluated. The medications that they are evaluated on, a plan is developed with that patient for the management of their pain that would again lead to the least risky, most effective way of managing their pain.

Chairman SANDERS. I want to thank all of our panelists. This Committee considers the issue of overmedication to be a serious national problem, a problem within the VA and a problem within the DOD. We appreciate your focusing on it and the good work you are doing. So, thank you all very much.

At this time I want to introduce our second panel. First, I am pleased to welcome Dr. Janet Kahn, who is a member of the Department of Psychiatry at the University of Vermont and Senior Policy Adviser for the Consortium of Academic Health Centers for Integrative Medicine. That is a mouthful.

Then we have Dr. Mark Edlund, who is the Senior Research Public Health Analyst in the Behavioral Health Epidemiology Program at RTI International.

Thank you both very much for being with us.

Dr. Kahn, let us begin with you.

STATEMENT OF JANET KAHN, Ph.D., RESEARCH ASSISTANT PROFESSOR, DEPARTMENT OF PSYCHIATRY, UNIVERSITY OF VERMONT AND SENIOR POLICY ADVISOR, CONSORTIUM OF ACADEMIC HEALTH CENTERS FOR INTEGRATIVE MEDICINE

Ms. KAHN. Chairman Sanders, Ranking Member Burr, Members of the Committee, I want to thank you for the honor of testifying before this distinguished body on what we all agree is a really critical issue, the issue of overmedication, particularly overuse of opioids for pain management.

I have been asked to share my understanding of what integrative health care approaches could offer to people in pain and people treating them.

So, by way of background, I am a medical sociologist and for the past 30 years my work has focused on issues of integrative health care. I am also a clinician. I am a massage therapist and instructor of meditation and somatic awareness training. So, in that capacity in the treatment room what I have spent the last 30 years doing is trying to understand how people can move from illness to wellness, from pain and ease, and how a nervous system that has gotten stuck in a flight or fight or freeze state can reset itself for optimal functioning.

For the past 5 years, almost all of my work has been with veterans of OEF, OIF, and OND and their partners. I have seen them in my private practice; and with my research partner, William Collinge, we utilize a program called Mission Reconnect.

This is a self-directed, home-use Web- and app-based program that offers instructions to help veterans and their partners learn various mind-body techniques that we know to support mental, physical, and relationship health.

Preliminary research that was conducted with veterans of the Vermont and Oregon National Guard units showed 8 weeks of this program to be effective in decreasing pain, decreasing anxiety levels, and decreasing people scores on PTSD checklist measurements.

We are now conducting a randomized clinical trial of Mission Reconnect in San Diego, Dallas, Fayetteville, North Carolina, and New York to understand the regional differences and to cover all branches of the military.

The term "integrative medicine" has been used with various meanings, so, I want to be clear that when I speak of integrative health care, I use the term to refer to team-based, coordinated use of the most appropriate evidence-based interventions from across the full conventional, complementary, and alternative medicine spectrum, including preventive efforts and a particular focus on interventions that educate and engage the patient and his or her family members in their own care and, therefore, hopefully leaving them with skills for a lifetime.

I think we all know the relevant reports from the Army Pain Management Task Force and the IOM, and I would like to echo those reports in calling for a comprehensive change not only in how we treat pain but literally how we think about pain so that it can guide the treatment beginning with understanding that we do not actually treat pain, we treat people in all their complexity, and pain is part of what they bring to the picture.

So many of the men and women returning from these wars have multiple wounds. They have injuries to their bodies, to their brains, to their hearts, to their minds, to their spirits, to their relationships; and we need to find a way to deal with that complexity as we treat them because they need more than just having their symptoms quieted. They actually need help learning to heal and to lead fulfilling lives in the many decades, being young, that they have ahead of them.

Our current approach to pain management can too easily lead to prescribing a drug for each identified problem and that in turn, as we know, can lead to a poly pharmacy problem that we may not have the capacity to actually manage.

These veterans have already been asked to carry and maneuver with more weight in their packs than their bodies were designed for. They have been exposed to more stress than their nervous systems can manage as we see absolutely every day. So, over medicating them is no solution and no gift.

There are evidence-based, non-pharmaceutical ways to address pain. In this kind of complexity, I suggest that we reorient toward a positive vision of health and wellness for our veterans; try to come up under them.

We know that lack of sleep, emotional stress, inability to take a deep breath, these things exacerbate pain. They literally make pain hurt more. They change the experience of it.

So, addressing the building blocks of wellness can reduce the need for pain medication, and research clearly indicates that massage, acupuncture, yoga, and other mind-body therapies can significantly enhance sleep quality as well as duration, can help the nervous system rest down and thus reduce the experience of physical and emotional pain and alter the treatment needs for it.

Educational interventions that include family members or groups of veterans can impart needed skills at the same time that they build community; and loss of community is an important element of a veteran's pain.

So, on top of all that they have already offered this country, veterans are offering us, I believe, the opportunity to embrace a wellness approach to the care of people who have incurred complex trauma, to kick our pharmaceuticals-only habit, come up with something more complex and interactive, and learn to collaborate across disciplines on their behalf. We should recognize this as one more gift they are giving us and move toward it quickly.

[The prepared statement of Ms. Kahn follows:]

TESTIMONY OF JANET KAHN, PH.D., RESEARCH ASSISTANT PROFESSOR, DEPARTMENT OF PSYCHIATRY, UNIVERSITY OF VERMONT AND SENIOR POLICY ADVISOR, CONSORTIUM OF ACADEMIC HEALTH CENTERS FOR INTEGRATIVE MEDICINE

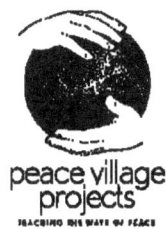

peace village
projects
TEACHING THE WAYS OF PEACE

Janet R. Kahn, PhD, EdM, LMT

Invited Testimony

United States Senate
Committee on Veterans' Affairs
Senator Bernie Sanders, Chairman
Senator Richard Burr, Ranking Member

April 30, 2014

Chairman Sanders, Ranking Member Burr and Members of the Committee:

Thank you for the honor to testify before this distinguished body regarding how best to serve our veterans, who as we all know, face enormous physical and emotional challenges. The issue that prompts this hearing, overmedication of our veterans, as well as active duty service members and civilians, particularly overuse of opioids for pain management, is a critical one. I have been asked to share my understanding of what integrative healthcare approaches might offer to people in pain.

By way of background, I am a social scientist, a medical sociologist. For the past 30 years my research and policy-oriented work have focused on integrative health care. I am also a clinician – a massage therapist, and an instructor in meditation and somatic awareness. For these same thirty years, in the treatment room, I have sought to understand what helps people move from illness to wellness, from pain to ease; and how a nervous system that has become stuck in a fight or flight or freeze response, can reset itself for optimal functioning.

For the past five years I have worked with Veterans of OIF/OEF/OND and their partners. I have seen them in my private practice, and with my research partner, William Collinge, have developed a program called Mission Reconnect. This is a self-directed, home use, web and app-based program, offering instruction to both veterans and their partners in a number of mind-body practices that support mental, physical and relationship health. Preliminary research, conducted with Veterans from Vermont and Oregon National Guard units showed 8-weeks of this program to be effective in decreasing pain, anxiety and PTSD scores.[1] We are now conducting an NIMH-funded large randomized clinical trial in four cities, with veterans from all branches of the military.

---

[1] Collinge W, Kahn J, Soltysik R. Promoting Reintegration of National Guard Veterans and Their Partners Using a Self-Directed Program of Integrative Therapies: A Pilot Study. *Military Medicine*, December 2012, vol. 177, no. 12, pp. 1477-1485(9)

The United States has a drug problem. In our veteran, active duty and civilian populations we face an enormous public health crisis of chronic pain, which must be addressed without creating a second problem of overuse of prescription and over the counter medications. Many have noticed this problem. The 2010 report of the Army Pain Management Task Force, chartered by Army Surgeon General Schoomaker, and the 2012 Institute of Medicine (IOM) report entitled *"Relieving Pain in America: A Blueprint for Transforming Prevention, Care, Education, and Research"* each in their own way call for a cultural transformation in our understanding and treatment of pain. The Task Force Report specifically called for first, an unprecedented level of coordination between the Military Health System and the Veterans Health Administration; and secondly, for the use of complementary and alternative therapies along with conventional medical approaches.

I join that call for a comprehensive change in how we think about and treat pain, beginning with the understanding that our job is to treat people, whole people in all their complexity – pain being part of what they bring to the picture. I support the broad implementation of patient-centered integrative health care, by which I mean team-based coordinated use of the most appropriate proven therapies, products and approaches from across the conventional, complementary and alternative medicine spectrum, including a strong focus on interventions that educate and engage the patient and his or her family members. That is the summary statement. Now a few words on why we need integrative health care and some challenges to its implementation.

We have a tsunami of need returning home from these wars - young people with multiple wounds – injuries to their bodies and their brains, as well as to their minds, hearts and spirits. The veterans I see need not just to be fixed up and have their symptoms quieted. They need help to heal, to live fulfilling lives. They have decades ahead of them. A reductionist approach of addressing each specific injury, each location of pain, each troublesome symptom, will not do. Thinking of each source of pain in isolation and prescribing a drug specifically for it, too easily leads to polypharmacy effects beyond our capacity to predict or manage. These people have already been asked to carry and maneuver with more weight in their pack than their bodies were designed for; they have already experienced more stress than their nervous systems can manage and we see the results of that every day. Overmedicating them is no solution. I hear from veterans increasingly, their suspicion that the suicides of their friends are at least in part a result of depression and confusion arising from too many medications. I don't know if they are right.

I do know that emotional and physical pain are inter-related in people, and that there are evidence-based non-pharmaceutical ways to address these that we should deploy. Wayne Jonas and colleagues at the Samueli Institute have coined the term "war-related trauma spectrum response" to capture the reality that veterans' experience of the impact of their multiple injuries cuts across the boundaries of anatomy, biology, neurology, psychology, and that our responses to them must be comparably holistic and integrative.[2]

Many complementary and alternative medicine therapies also cross these boundaries in their effects. Acupuncture used to be spoken of entirely in terms of energy or chi. Yet, research by my colleague at the University of Vermont, Dr. Helene Langevin, has shown that when a thin acupuncture needle is inserted, collagen fibers from the connective tissue adhere to the needle, which prompts a stretch in the fascia, which in turn, prompts certain gene expression, and the

---

[2] Jonas W, et al. Acupuncture for the Trauma Spectrum Response: Scientific Foundations, Challenges to Implementation, Medical Acupuncture, 2011, vol.23, no. 4, pp.249-262.

chain of effect continues leading to effects that touch many aspects of the person and endure well beyond the duration of needle insertion. [3] Therapeutic massage is often regarded as a physical medicine, but research shows that it produces EEG changes, specifically increased frontal delta power and decreased frontal alpha and theta power – a combination correlated with simultaneous relaxation and alertness – a relatively pleasant and helpful state of mind.[4]

We need to re-orient toward a positive vision of health and wellness for our veterans, not just approach them with a problem-fixing mentality. Sufficient high-quality sleep, appropriate nutrition, compassionate touch whether from a human friend or a therapy dog, experience of community and a sense of purpose are all factors in human well-being. Lack of sleep, emotional stress, and the inability to take a deep breath – these things exacerbate our experience of physical pain. They literally make pain hurt more. Addressing these building blocks of wellness can reduce the need for pain medication. Research clearly indicates that massage, acupuncture, yoga and other mind-body therapies can significantly enhance sleep quality, help the nervous system rest down, and thus reduce physical and emotional pain. Educational interventions that include family members or groups of veterans can impart needed skills at the same time that they build community. Loss of community is a real source of pain for many veterans post-deployment.

There will be challenges in making this change. I will name three. First is the hegemony of pharmaceuticals in conventional medicine's approach to pain treatment and in the US in general. The pharmaceutical industry is heavily invested in drugs being the first thought of every provider and patient, and thus we see them advertised on television every day. It will take a conscious decision to bring other proven approaches into the mix. In contrast, educational tools offering veterans a lifetime of help in their own self-care cost very little to put into every home. No one profits from them financially. Thus they are not advertised as are pharmaceuticals. It is our responsibility to bring them prominently into the picture.

Second, we all need a big dose of humility, and support in relinquishing professional territoriality. If any health care profession were already responding satisfactorily to the multi-dimensional needs our veterans are living with, you would not have called this hearing. Integration requires real teamwork. Teamwork requires humility and mutual respect. We must respect not only one another's therapies, but also the fact that both reductionis and holistic thinking will contribute to best care.

Third, the VA is a big system and big systems are hard to change. But the VA also has a compelling purpose, strong leadership and a stated commitment to patient-centered care and cultural transformation. It is also a true single system – unlike the rest of US healthcare, so it is ideally suited to lead the way.

People are complex, integrated, and highly individual beings. Our treatment approaches need to match this. On top of all they have already offered this country, veterans are offering us the opportunity to embrace a wellness approach to the care of people who have incurred complex trauma, to kick our pharmaceuticals only habit of medicine and to learn to collaborate across disciplines, on their behalf. We should recognize this as one more gift from them and move forward as quickly as we responsibly can.

---

[3] Langevin HM, The Science of Stretch, *The Scientist*, May1, 2013

[4] Field T, et al; Massage therapy reduces anxiety and enhances EEG pattern of alertness and math computations, *Int J Neurosci.* 1996 Sep;86(3-4):197-205.

Published in final edited form as:
Mil Med. 2012 December ; 177(12): 1477–1485.

Promoting Reintegration of National Guard Veterans and Their Partners Using a Self-Directed Program of Integrative Therapies: A Pilot Study

William Collinge, MPH, PhD[*], **Janet Kahn, PhD, LMT**[†], and **Robert Soltysik, MS**[‡]

[*]Collinge and Associates, 3986 N Shasta Loop, Eugene, OR 97405

[†]Peace Village Projects, Inc., 240 Maple St, Burlington, VT 05401

[‡]213 N St SE, Glen Burnie, MD 21061

Abstract

This article reports pilot data from phase I of a project to develop and evaluate a self-directed program of integrative therapies for National Guard personnel and significant relationship partners to support reintegration and resilience after return from Iraq or Afghanistan. Data are reported on 43 dyads. Intervention was an integrated multimedia package of guided meditative, contemplative, and relaxation exercises (CD) and instruction in simple massage techniques (DVD) to promote stress reduction and interpersonal connectedness. A repeated measures design with standardized instruments was used to establish stability of baseline levels of relevant mental health domains (day 1, day 30), followed by the intervention and assessments 4 and 8 weeks later. Significant improvements in standardized measures for post-traumatic stress disorder, depression, and self-compassion were seen in both veterans and partners; and in stress for partners. Weekly online reporting tracked utilization of guided exercises and massage. Veterans reported significant reductions in ratings of physical pain, physical tension, irritability, anxiety/worry, and depression after massage, and longitudinal analysis suggested declining baseline levels of tension and irritability. Qualitative data from focus groups and implications for continued development and a phase II trial are discussed.

INTRODUCTION

Psychological distress and adjustment difficulties among military veterans returning from Operation Iraqi Freedom (OIF) and Operation Enduring Freedom (OEF) and their relationship partners are well documented.[1–3] Screening efforts suggest that up to 42% of National Guard veterans and roughly one-third of all returning veterans have problems that warrant mental health treatment, yet most are not receiving treatment. Many returnees express concerns about interpersonal conflict, highlighting the potential impact of deployment-related psychological distress on the well-being of veterans' family members, friends, and coworkers.[3,4]

Perceived stigma associated with seeking behavioral health services remains a barrier to needed treatment.[5] Sayer et al[6] reported both individual and sociocultural barriers cited by veterans as reasons for not seeking treatment. With the numbers of veterans that will be reintegrating into community life in the coming years, the long-term impact of untreated or undertreated mental health problems is expected to impact communities for years to come.

As a distinct population, members of the National Guard face circumstances different from those of veterans of other branches of the military in terms of access to services during reintegration. Rather than returning to a base that may offer a comprehensive range of services and the camaraderie of others who have shared their experiences, they return to their home communities as "citizen soldiers." Although eligible for Veterans Administration (VA) benefits, distance to VA facilities and Vet Centers may pose an obstacle that limits their use of those opportunities, particularly in rural states. Although other veterans who return to a base spend their days among those who recognize their service, rank, and experiences, and may also be alert to signals of mental difficulties, National Guard veterans returning to prior jobs may well be earning less pay, having less responsibility, and receiving less respect from coworkers who have never experienced them in their military capacities. From a community health perspective, National Guard veterans are a population at significant risk of being underserved in terms of mental health needs. Thus, innovative interventions that overcome the psychological, geographical, and financial obstacles to accessing formal services and help this population reintegrate and adjust to community life in the long term are needed. Of particular interest are interventions that target maladaptive coping strategies commonly addressed in cognitive behavioral interventions such as worry, self-punishment, and social avoidance, and that bolster social support as these may reduce combat-related symptoms in this population.[7]

This article reports pilot data from a phase I National Institute of Mental Health–funded study of a behavioral health intervention designed for autonomous use at home by National Guard veterans and partners of their choice to promote reintegration and well-being. The project is entitled "Mission Reconnect: Promoting Resilience and Reintegration of Post-Deployment Veterans and Their Families." The intervention, delivered by CD, DVD, and print, integrates instruction in evidence-based complementary therapies supporting both individual and relationship well-being. The program is designed to be self-directed with its different elements used at home, at work, or anywhere the participant finds them helpful. People may use each element of the program as frequently or infrequently as they like. Using it requires neither travel to VA or other facilities nor labeling oneself as in need of mental health care. The wellness-oriented techniques in this program are appropriate for people across a broad spectrum of mental health status and may be used by themselves or as an adjunct to individual or group therapies. Thus, the program may be able to reach people who are geographically isolated from services as well as people who are reluctant to use mental health services.

Mission Reconnect includes meditative, contemplative, and relaxation techniques and use of touch with a partner in the form of simple massage. Hundreds of small clinical trials indicate that mindfulness-related practices may offer significant benefits for a broad spectrum of health and mental health outcomes including stress, depression, and post-traumatic stress disorder (PTSD), including with military populations.[8–10] However, given the size and quality of these studies (many, for instance, lacked plausible comparison groups), their findings must be taken as suggestive rather than definitive. A recent systematic review of complementary and alternative medicine (CAM) therapies for depressive and anxiety disorders concluded that "For anxiety disorders, there is limited evidence on the effectiveness of meditation (n = 2 studies).... Relaxation and/or breathing retraining show promise as a CAM therapy.... Mindfulness-based stress reduction has shown positive effects on anxiety and depressive symptoms. However, studies are poor to fair quality."[11] Other systematic reviews have drawn similar conclusions.

The literature on massage is somewhat stronger, with massage methods, including simple relaxation massage, having been established as beneficial for a broad spectrum of conditions, with reductions in anxiety and pain among the most common benefits.[12–18]

While using these often-studied techniques, this investigation breaks new ground in part by delivering the instruction solely through self-directed media. In our own prior research, we

68

found not only that people are able to learn simple touch and massage techniques from video with no personal instruction but also that the resulting massages produced reductions of pain, fatigue, anxiety, and depression, on a par with those of professional massage therapists.[19] Although mind–body techniques are now taught in many medical schools,[20] and their use is fairly widespread, we found no research on the effects of these techniques when taught exclusively by CD and/or audiotape even though tapes and CDs teaching mind–body techniques are ubiquitous. Although both massage and mind–body techniques are increasingly used in VA and Department of Defense sites around the country, our program's emphasis on self-directed media delivery of instruction is, to our knowledge, novel for the military population.

A key aspect of this program is targeting the dyadic system of a veteran and trusted partner for intervention. As stated in the Iraq War Clinician Guide, "The primary source of support for the returning soldier is likely to be his or her family. We know from veterans of the Vietnam War that there can be a risk of disengagement from family at the time of return from a war zone. We also know that emerging problems with ASD (acute stress disorder) and PTSD can wreak havoc with the competency and comfort the returning soldier experiences as a partner and parent."[21]

Although it is clear that formal mental health support is warranted for a large number of returning veterans, the people in their significant relationships are seriously affected as well.[22–27] Early support for both the veteran and family may increase the potential for successful reintegration and family cohesion and reduce the likelihood or severity of future problems. Thus, the goal of Mission Reconnect is to offer an integrated program that leverages the relationship bond to encourage compliance, teaches stress-management skills to both the veteran and partner, and strengthens the relationship through joint use of wellness-related practices and guidance in generating compassion and appreciation for self and partner. This article reports on a phase I feasibility study of the approach.

METHODS

Recruitment and Sample

Recruitment was conducted with the cooperation of the Family Support and Assistance Programs (FSAPs) of the Army National Guard in both Vermont and Oregon. Subjects were recruited through presentations at postdeployment Yellow Ribbon events and through announcement in FSAP e-newsletters. Subjects were consented in person or by phone by the first author, and institutional review board oversight was provided by the New England Institutional Review Board, Newton, Massachusetts.

Baseline Phase

Subjects completed a 30-day baseline phase (no intervention) with survey data (described below) collected at the beginning (baseline 1) and end of the 30 period (baseline 2) to establish stability of baseline levels on standardized instruments (see the section "Data Collection").

Intervention Phase

Intervention began with a 2-hour orientation meeting in which subjects were given the intervention package (CD, DVD, manual, described below), viewed the materials as a group, and received instructions for home practice and data collection.

Intervention activities were of two types: (1) mind/body practices (meditative, contemplative, and relaxation techniques) taught by audio CD and print instruction and (2) massage for stress reduction (taught by video DVD and print/photographic instruction). Subjects were instructed to practice their choice of practices at least 3 to 4 times per week for 8 weeks and to try them all at least once during the course of the 8-week intervention period.

For massage, we instructed the subjects to practice massage techniques of their choice as often as they mutually agreed each week, suggesting that they may benefit from sessions of just a few minutes on up to 30 minutes or more. This would allow us to collect data on preferences and utilization patterns. In addition to these general instructions, we asked all dyads to do one 20-minute session per week as a "massage reporting session." This would allow us to collect data on change in veterans' symptoms after a uniform dose of partner-delivered massage across the sample. (This weekly reporting session was not assumed to be representative of all sessions because of expected variations in duration.) We used this approach successfully in a prior study for assessing the ability of caregivers to provide relief through massage at home.[19]

Data Collection

All data were collected online via PsychData.com. Data were collected both monthly and weekly. The monthly survey package was administered to both veterans and partners at baselines 1 and 2 (30 days apart), 4 weeks after beginning intervention, and again at 8 weeks (end of intervention). We used the PTSD Checklist—Civilian Version (PCL-C)[28] for both the veteran and the partner. The PCL-C is a 17-item self-report scale that assesses the Diagnostic and Statistical Manual for Mental Disorders (Edition 4) diagnostic symptoms of PTSD using a Likert-type response format. It has demonstrated excellent internal consistency and test-retest reliability and correlates highly with other measures of PTSD.[29] The PCL-C is used rather than the PCL-Military because it is important to assess veterans' responses to military and nonmilitary traumatic events. The PCL-C was used with partners and veterans since partners of veterans with PTSD may experience secondary trauma stress;[30,31] veterans with PTSD have increased tendency toward intimate partner violence,[32] and women who have experienced intimate partner violence have increased incidence of PTSD.[33,34] The incidence of PTSD among partners of OIF/OEF veterans remains understudied.

To assess depression, we used the Beck Depression Inventory II (BDI-II). This is one of the most widely used instruments for measuring depression and uses a 21-item scale with reliability and validity established in numerous studies. Respondents are asked to rate their symptoms and attitudes using a 4-point scale. Normative values for a variety of patient populations are available as reliability figures,[35] and comparison data on OIF veterans are provided in the section "Results."

Subjects completed the Perceived Stress Scale (PSS-10), a 10-item Likert-scaled instrument to determine perceived stress levels over a 1-month recall period. The PSS is a validated and widely used scale for community samples with at least a junior high school education. The items are general in nature and free of content specific to any subpopulation group.[36]

To assess capacity for compassion toward others, we used the Compassionate Love Scale ("Close Other" version), 21 items with a single score that assesses compassionate or altruistic love. Studies with three samples ($N = 529$) were used to create the scale that was tested in three new studies ($N = 700$) for validation and to identify correlates of compassionate love. Correlates were seen with indices of prosocial behavior such as helping others, social support to close others, and empathy with others ($a = 0.95$).[37]

We also used the Self-Compassion Scale, a 26-item, 5-point Likert measure of 6 different aspects of self-compassion: self-kindness, self-judgment, common humanity, isolation, mindfulness, and overidentification. The scale has an appropriate factor structure and demonstrates concurrent validity (e.g., correlates with social connectedness), convergent validity (e.g., correlates with lower anxiety, depression, and perfectionism, and greater satisfaction with life), discriminate validity (e.g., no correlation with social desirability or narcissism and appears to promote better coping than self-esteem),[38,39] and test–retest reliability ($\alpha = 0.93$).[40]

To assess quality of life, we used the Quality of Life Inventory (QoLI),[41] a 32-item questionnaire with evidence for concurrent, discriminant, predictive, and criterion-related validity. It includes subscales for health, self-esteem, goals and values, money, work, play, learning, creativity, helping, love, friends, children, relatives, home, neighborhood, and community and an overall score. It was validated in a study involving 3,927 clients from various clinical settings and has been found sensitive to treatment-related change in naturalistic clinical settings and samples.[42]

In addition to the above monthly survey instruments, both veteran and partner submitted a weekly report online each week during the 8-week intervention phase. The weekly reports recorded (1) frequency and duration of use of each intervention method offered plus (2) data from both the veteran and partner specific to the massage reporting session. Massage session data for the veteran comprised pre- and postsession ratings (recorded at time of massage on a two-sided, 5 × 8-inch session card) for levels of physical pain, physical tension, irritability, anxiety/worry, and depression, each rated for severity on a 0 to 10 scale. Massage data for the partner comprised areas of the body massaged and duration of the reporting session. All session card data were later entered by the subjects individually on their online weekly report.

Subject compensation was $20 for each weekly report and $25 for each monthly survey.

Instructional Materials

Video Instruction—A DVD was professionally produced with the following contents: (a) Introduction to Mission Reconnect by LTC Wayne Jonas, MD (Ret.), U.S. Army Medical Corps (welcoming and endorsing the program, 2:15), (b) Overview of the Project (W.C., purpose and goals, 1:45), A Word on PTSD (W.C., responding if symptoms arise during exercises, 1:21), How to Participate (W.C., setting aside time daily for wellness practices, willingness to test practices, 0:50), The Tools (W.C., types of practices, frequency and duration of use, 1:05), and (c) Instruction in Massage for Stress Reduction (J.K., overview, communication, preparation, affirming nonsexual intention; instruction in light massage techniques for the head and face, neck, shoulders, back, feet, and hands, using home furniture, 29:00).

Audio Instruction—The first two authors (W.C., J.K.) produced and recorded an audio CD with the following guided mind/body practices: "Centering" (basic mindfulness meditation instruction, 11:36, male and female voice versions), "Connecting" (contemplative guided meditation to encourage appreciation, compassion, and well-wishing for the partner and self, 7:03, male and female voice versions), "Deep Relaxation" (progressive relaxation through the body, 20:12, male voice), "Sound Into Silence" (following the tone of a struck chime into silence to facilitate meditative state, 4:16, female voice), "Movement Into Stillness" (seated, gentle rocking in progressively reduced movements until still, 5:32, female voice), and "Therapeutic Yawning" (evocation of the yawning reflex for a series of six to twelve yawns, 3:16, female voice). Subjects were

71

encouraged to download the exercises to their mobile devices for practice any time of day they wished (though we did not collect data on devices used).

Printed Manual—The project manual (47 pages) includes the text of the introductory DVD material, descriptions and specific instructions for each of the guided mind/body exercises, and instructions for the massage techniques accompanied by photos.

Follow-Up Focus Groups

A convenience sample of 12 dyads (self-selected), who were able to attend at the scheduled meeting times, participated in two 90-minute follow-up focus groups after the completion of intervention. The purpose was to provide qualitative data on perceived impact of the program, usability of the materials, and recommendations for future development. The meetings were recorded, transcribed, and analyzed using QSR NVivo software for thematic analysis and coding of participant comments. Participants were compensated $50 for attendance.

Deployment-Related Interruption

Hurricane Irene struck New England roughly midway through the intervention phase for the Vermont cohort, requiring temporary deployment of some subjects. Given study's primary goal of assessing feasibility of the instructional approach, we decided to accommodate this by instructing affected dyads to pause their weekly reporting regimes until after the soldier returned so as to have 8 weeks of complete data from participating dyads. We address this further in the section "Discussion."

RESULTS

Sample

Forty-three dyads were consented (27 Vermont, 16 Oregon). Of these, 23 veterans had 1 deployment, 18 had 2 deployments, and 2 had 3 deployments; 8 were OIF only, 20 OEF only, and 15 had been in both OIF and OEF. The sample includes service members with return dates ranging from 2002 to 2011. As seen in Figure 1, of 43 consented dyads, 41 provided baseline data, 38 began intervention, and 32 completed the final follow-up (84% of intervention starters). Demographics of the sample are shown in Table I. In all cases of dropout for which we were able to attain information, reasons given were related to time commitment involved to do project activities.

Fidelity

Subjects averaged over six times per week using one or more of the mind/body exercises and more than 2.5 times using massage (Table II); thus, for both modalities, fidelity exceeded the minimum instructions. Minutes per week devoted to both modalities combined averaged 61 for veterans and 63.3 for partners.

Mind/Body Practices

Of mind/body exercises, the Therapeutic Yawning, Centering, and Deep Relaxation exercises were most used. Subjects reported using the mind/body practices an average of 6.3 times per week; veterans averaged 27 minutes (SD 17.6), and partners 27.6 minutes (SD 15.6).

Massage Data

Mean duration of the 136 massage reporting sessions conducted was 22.7 minutes (SD 5.5), and the most prominent areas massaged were shoulders (75%), neck (72%), back (68%), head (36%), and feet (27%). Veterans reported highly significant reductions after massage for physical pain, physical tension, irritability, anxiety/worry, and depression (Table III). Change over time in veterans' presession ratings of symptom levels was analyzed by splitting each veteran's weekly reporting sessions into an early series and a late series, and then comparing the two series using Kendall's tau-b (Table IV). Significant declines were seen over time in presession ratings for "physical tension" and "on edge/irritable."

Survey Data

For all survey instruments, two baseline testings showed no significant differences; thus, the mean scores of two baseline testings were calculated for each subject for reporting as their "baseline" (Table V).

Post-Traumatic Stress Disorder—Baseline scores for veterans on the PCL-C (mean 34.7, SD 13.6) were close to those of a study of 355 OIF veterans by Erbes et al[43] (mean 35.5, SD 13.6, using the Military version of the PCL). The VA National Center for PTSD suggests cutoffs for screening and diagnostic purposes,[44] with a screening cutoff of 25 for both active duty OIF/OEF veterans and civilians and diagnostic cutoffs of 28 and 30 to 38, respectively.[45–47] Thus, there appeared to be substantial risk of PTSD in both veterans and partners in our sample, and both veterans and partners showed significant, though modest, improvements at both follow-ups.

Depression—Baseline depression scores for veterans (mean 12.6, SD 11.5) were higher than that of Erbes et al sample (mean 9.78, SD 7.95). The cutoffs used for the BDI-II are 0 to 9 for minimal depression, 10 to 16 for mild, 17 to 29 for moderate, and 30 to 63 for severe. Both veterans and partners showed significant reductions from the mild range to the minimal range at follow-up.

Other Scales—The PSS-10, Compassionate Love Scale, and Self-Compassion Scale are not diagnostic instruments, so there are no cutoffs. Partners showed significant reductions in perceived stress, and both partners and veterans had significant improvements in self-compassion at first follow-up and a trend at second follow-up. There were no significant changes on the Compassionate Love Scale, although over half of the subjects improved their scores at both follow-ups. The QoLI showed no significant outcomes on any subscales or total score. Those data are not presented here but are available on request.

Qualitative Data (From Focus Groups)

Participants reported practicing the exercises at home, at work, and in their vehicles. They viewed the project and each of its elements as well designed and beneficial. They endorsed the inclusion of all the elements even though they individually selected elements that best suited their personalities and/or life circumstances: "Regardless of where I was during the day, I felt like I could use Centering when I felt things getting kind of edgy and unsettled." The overall program was described as providing useful ways of managing stress and improving their couple relationship: "...the Connecting, with thinking about what I appreciated in him, that was nothing new, but sharing it with him was a new piece and it helped me to open up more", and "I think it's a great post-deployment type thing, because you are so separate for so long, it definitely did draw us back towards each other..." The participants strongly endorsed the program and proposed its broader availability to veterans and families: "...the guys are under a lot of stress, and we are under a lot of stress at home, even without the deployment. The military world is a different world, so anything from this aspect of empowering themselves and couples is just great, so thanks for bringing it to us."

DISCUSSION

As noted in the section "Methods", some dyads had data collection interrupted for emergency deployment during Hurricane Irene. Given our primary goal of evaluating feasibility of the instructional approach, we deemed delayed reporting to be an appropriate, though imperfect, solution to obtain a full 8 weeks of "normal use" data. Nine dyads were affected. These partners and some veterans were free to practice to the extent they could during nonreported weeks (though some veterans were working 18–20 hours per day). Four dyads required an additional 2 weeks, 3 an additional 4 weeks, and 2 an additional 5 to 7 weeks to achieve 8 weeks of reporting. For these 9 dyads, we cannot rule out potential historical confounds, either negative (e.g., greater stress) or positive (e.g., more practice, maturation), affecting their monthly survey data.

One of the most important findings of this pilot study concerns compliance/fidelity. We found that postdeployment National Guard veterans and their partners were able and willing to follow the recommended utilization of the proposed health promotion activities. Williams et al, in a review of CAM therapies that they conducted for the VA, found that the studies they reviewed often reported high rates of dropout. From this, they concluded that adherence to meditation may be problematic in a clinical setting. Although our methods do not allow a direct comparison to these studies, it appears that our adherence may have been higher, perhaps because of the support of the partner relationship.

This also contrasts with the often-lamented avoidance of help seeking or self-help commonly attributed to the military population. We observed during recruitment that most dyads entering the study were led by the partner initiating the contact (e.g., bringing the soldier to our table at a Yellow Ribbon event or telling their soldier "we need this" in response to a newsletter announcement). This affirms the viability, indeed the importance, of leveraging an existing trusted relationship as a strategy for engaging the veteran in health-promoting reintegration activity. Also, although we offered the project to veteran/partner dyads of all kinds, including parent/adult, child, sibling or friend, only one dyad entered the study that was not a spouse/life partner relationship. It appears that inclusion of massage, although deemed very helpful by those who participated in Mission Reconnect, calls for a level of intimacy that may not be seen as suitable by this population for other types of relationships. A somewhat different approach needs to be explored for nonpartnered veterans.

The data on massage for veterans suggest that partners may achieve significant acute effects for veterans' stress-related symptoms with minimal instruction in very basic massage techniques. Perhaps, more striking was the finding that preseason levels of most symptoms declined over time, suggesting declining background levels of most symptoms over the intervention period for veterans. Although post-massage ratings can be attributed to the massage, change in premassage ratings over time cannot be attributed to a single source with confidence. Participants reported during focus groups that they felt the whole program was beneficial in symptom reduction and relationship strengthening, but with no comparison group, we cannot be certain how much of their increased comfort is program effect or simply a matter of time and settling in, so to speak. This will be tested in phase II.

Although data were not collected on effects of veteran-delivered massage on partners in follow-up focus groups, there was consensus that partners wanted and appreciated receiving massage and that veterans found satisfaction in providing it. This was an unanticipated finding that we will explore further in phase II as potentially supportive of reintegration and relationship quality.

Collinge et al.

The survey data suggest that the intervention approach may yield significant reductions during the reintegration process, for both veterans and their partners, in measures of PTSD, stress, depression, and self-compassion. Depression scores (BDI-II) for both veterans and partners dropped from the mild range to the minimal range during intervention. Mean PTSD scores were below the threshold for the clinical diagnosis (50) from baseline onward, though a substantial range in scores was seen. The change in self-compassion scores is of particular interest in light of the concept of "moral injury" as related to PTSD in OIF/OEF veterans.[48] The absence of significant change on the Compassionate Love Scale may be because of a ceiling effect, given that baseline scores were relatively close to the maximum possible score (105). The lack of significant effects on the QoLI may be a function of insufficient sensitivity of the instrument or too small a sample.

Finally, we recognize that reintegration and resilience are multifaceted constructs. In this feasibility study, we sought to assess potential for impact of the intervention on some variables that theoretically contribute to those broad constructs. In phase II, with feasibility established, we will focus more directly on measures of both reintegration and resilience, as well as sleep and relationship quality, in a four-armed randomized controlled trial. We plan to refine the intervention approach based on phase I data; use web-based delivery to computers and mobile devices so that it can be a fully autonomous, self-directed intervention; and then compare outcomes to a standard of care in-person program currently being used in the military to promote reintegration and resilience.

CONCLUSIONS

Veterans and their partners in this sample showed willingness to engage and use the mind/body practices and massage methods offered in Mission Reconnect and appeared to benefit from them. This study suggests that leveraging a trusted relationship may offer a viable approach to implementing self-directed interventions such as this for promoting well-being during postdeployment reintegration. Given that members of this branch of military are at particular risk for being underserved, in both short-term and long-term mental health service needs, autonomous and self-directed interventions may play an increasingly important role over time.

These pilot data encourage further development of the approach followed by testing with a larger and more diverse sample as is planned for phase II. Questions remaining to be answered include optimal duration of intervention period, longevity of effects, usability of the intervention by more ethnically diverse populations, and effects for veterans from various branches of the military.

Acknowledgments

The authors acknowledge the following whose support helped make this project possible: Lt Col Lloyd Goodrow, Col Jon Coffin, the staff of the Family Support and Assistance Program, veterans and family members of the Vermont National Guard; Michelle Kochosky, Jennifer Kotz and Chaplain Daniel Thompson of the Oregon National Guard Family Program, veterans and family members; Wayne B. Jonas, MD, LTC USA MC (Ret.), and Executive Director, The Samueli Institute; Melissa Paly and Bill Rogers of Cross Current Communications, Portsmouth, NH; Venerable Dhyani Ywahoo, Dr. Julio Henderson and Dr. Joanna Muoy, each of whose work provided important inspiration for Mission Reconnect; and Shiri Weaver, PhD, who conducted the qualitative analysis of focus group recordings. This project is funded by National Institute of Mental Health SBIR (Small Business Innovation Research) Grant No. R43MH088063 to Collinge and Associates.

References

1. Wells TS, Miller SC, Adler AB, Engel CC, Smith TC, Fairbank JA. Mental health impact of the Iraq and Afghanistan conflicts: a review of US research, service provision, and programmatic responses. Int Rev Psychiatry. 2011; 23(2):144–52. [PubMed: 21521083]

2. Otis JD, McGlinchey R, Vasterling JJ, Kerns RD. Complicating factors associated with mild traumatic brain injury: impact on pain and posttraumatic stress disorder treatment. J Clin Psychol Med Settings. 2011; 18(2):145–54. [PubMed: 21626354]

3. Tanielian, T.; Jaycox, LH. Psychological and Cognitive Injuries, Their Consequences and Services to Assist Recovery. Santa Monica, CA: Rand Center for Military Health Policy Research; 2008. Invisible Wounds of War; p. 453

4. Milliken CS, Auchterlonie JL, Hoge CW. Longitudinal assessment of mental health problems among active and reserve component soldiers returning from the Iraq war. JAMA. 2007; 298(18): 2141–8. [PubMed: 18000197]

5. Chiarelli, PW. Army Health Promotion, Risk Reduction, Suicide Prevention Report, 2010. Washington, DC: Headquarters, Department of the Army; 2010. Available at http://www.army.mil/article/42934

6. Sayer NA, Friedemann-Sanchez G, Spoont M, et al. A qualitative study of determinants of PTSD treatment initiation in veterans. Psychiatry. 2009; 72(3):238–55. [PubMed: 19821647]

7. Pietrzak RH, Harpaz-Rotem I, Southwick SM. Cognitive-behavioral coping strategies associated with combat related PTSD in treatment-seeking OEF-OIF Veterans. Psychiatry Res. 2011; 189(2): 251–8. [PubMed: 21813184]

8. Rees B. Overview of outcome data of potential meditation training for soldier resilience. Mil Med. 2011; 176(11):1232–42. [PubMed: 22165650]

9. Chiesa A. Vipassana meditation: systematic review of current evidence. J Altern Complement Med. 2010; 16(1):37–46. [PubMed: 20055558]

10. Cuellar NG. Mindfulness meditation for veterans—implications for occupational health providers. AAOHN J. 2008; 56(8):357–63. [PubMed: 18717302]

11. Williams, JW.; Gierisch, JM.; McDuffie, J.; Strauss, JL.; Nagi, A. Evidence-based Synthesis Program. Washington, DC: Health Services and Research and Development Service, Department of Veterans Affairs; 2011. An Overview of Complementary and Alternative Medicine Therapies for Anxiety and Depressive Disorders: Supplement to Efficacy of Complementary and Alternative Medicine Therapies for Posttraumatic Stress Disorder [Internet]. Available at http://www.ncbi.nlm.nih.gov/books/NBK82787

12. Hou WH, Chiang PT, Hsu TY, Chiu SY, Yen YC. Treatment effects of massage therapy in depressed people: a meta-analysis. J Clin Psychiatry. 2010; 71(7):894–901. [PubMed: 20361919]

13. Moyer CA, Rounds J, Hannum JW. A meta-analysis of massage therapy research. Psychol Bull. 2004; 130(1):3–18. [PubMed: 14717648]

14. McPherson F, Schwenka MA. Use of complementary and alternative therapies among active duty soldiers, military retirees, and family members at a military hospital. Mil Med. 2004; 169(5):354–7. [PubMed: 15185998]

15. Field T. Massage therapy. Med Clin North Am. 2002; 86(1):163–71. [PubMed: 11795087]

16. Field, T. Touch Therapy. New York: Churchill Livingston; 2000.

17. Field, T. Touch. Cambridge, MA: MIT Press; 2001.

18. Moraska A, Pollini RA, Boulanger K, Brooks MZ, Teitlebaum L. Physiological adjustments to stress measures following massage therapy: a review of the literature. Evid Based Complement Alternat Med. 2010; 7(4):409–18. [PubMed: 18955340]

19. Collinge W, Kahn J, Walton T, Fletcher K. Randomized controlled trial of family caregiver use of massage as supportive cancer care following multimedia instruction. J Soc Integr Oncol. 2009; 7(4):178.

20. Brokaw JJ, Tunnicliff G, Raess BU, Saxon DW. The teaching of complementary and alternative medicine in U.S. medical schools: a survey of course directors. Acad Med. 2002; 77(9):876–81. [PubMed: 12228082]

21. National Center for PTSD and Walter Reed Army Medical Center. Iraq War Clinician Guide. 2. National Center for PTSD; White River Junction, VT: 2004. p. 40Available at http://www.ptsd.va.gov/professional/manuals/iraq-war-clinician-guide.asp

22. Hayes J, Wakefield B, Andresen EM, et al. Identification of domains and measures for assessment battery to examine well-being of spouses of OIF/OEF veterans with PTSD. J Rehabil Res Dev. 2010; 47(9):825–40. [PubMed: 21174248]

23. Verdeli H, Baily C, Vousoura E, Belser A, Singla D, Manos G. The case for treating depression in military spouses. J Fam Psychol. 2011; 25(4):488–96. [PubMed: 21842994]

24. Mansfield AJ, Kaufman JS, Marshall SW, Gaynes BN. Morrissey JP, Engel CC. Deployment and the use of mental health services among U.S. Army wives. N Engl J Med. 2010; 362(2):101–9. [PubMed: 20071699]

25. Eaton KM, Hoge CW, Messer SC, et al. Prevalence of mental health problems, treatment need, and barriers to care among primary care-seeking spouses of military service members involved in Iraq and Afghanistan deployments. Mil Med. 2008; 173(11):1051–6. [PubMed: 19055177]

26. de Burgh HT, White CJ, Fear NT, Iversen AC. The impact of deployment to Iraq or Afghanistan on partners and wives of military personnel. Int Rev Psychiatry. 2011; 23(2):192–200. [PubMed: 21521089]

27. Calhoun PS, Beckham JC, Bosworth HB. Caregiver burden and psychological distress in partners of veterans with chronic posttraumatic stress disorder. J Trauma Stress. 2002; 15:205–12. [PubMed: 12092912]

28. Weathers, FW.; Huska, JA.; Keane, TM. PCL-C for DSM-IV. Boston, MA: Behavioral Science Division, National Center for PTSD; 1991.

29. Blanchard EB, Jones-Alexander J, Buckley TC, Forneris CA. Psychometric properties of the PTSD Checklist (PCL). Behav Res Ther. 1996; 34(8):669–73. [PubMed: 8870294]

30. Ein-Dor T, Doron G, Solomon Z, Mikulincer M, Shaver PR. Together in pain: attachment-related dyadic processes and posttraumatic stress disorder. J Couns Psychol. 2010; 57(3):317–27. [PubMed: 21133582]

31. Manguno-Mire G, Sautter F, Lyons J, et al. Psychological distress and burden among female partners of combat veterans with PTSD. J Nerv Ment Dis. 2007; 195(2):144–51. [PubMed: 17299302]

32. Hundt NE, Holohan DR. The role of shame in distinguishing perpetrators of intimate partner violence in U.S. veterans. J Trauma Stress. 2012; 25(2):191–7. [PubMed: 22522734]

33. Strigo IA, Simmons AN, Matthews SC, et al. Neural correlates of altered pain response in women with posttraumatic stress disorder from intimate partner violence. Biol Psychiatry. 2010; 68(5):442–50. [PubMed: 20553750]

34. Taft CT, Vogt DS, Mechanic MB, Resick PA. Posttraumatic stress disorder and physical health symptoms among women seeking help for relationship aggression. J Fam Psychol. 2007; 21(3):354–62. [PubMed: 17874920]

35. Beck, AT.; Steer, RA. Beck Depression Inventory Manual. San Antonio, TX: Harcourt Brace; 1993.

36. Cohen S, Kamarck T, Mermelstein R. A global measure of perceived stress. J Health Soc Behav. 1983; 24:385–96. [PubMed: 6668417]

37. Sprecher S, Fehr B. Compassionate love for close others and humanity. J Soc Pers Relat. 2005; 22:629–51.

38. Neff KD, Hsieh Y, Dejitterat K. Self-compassion, achievement goals, and coping with academic failure. Self and Identity. 2005; 4(3):263–87.

39. Neff KD, Rude SS, Kirkpatrick KL. An examination of self-compassion in relation to positive psychological functioning and personality traits. J Res Pers. 2007; 41:908–16.

40. Neff KD. The development and validation of a scale to measure self-compassion. Self and Identity. 2003; 2:223–50.

41. Frisch MB, Clark MP, Rouse SV, et al. Predictive and treatment validity of life satisfaction and the Quality of Life Inventory. Assessment. 2005; 12(1):66–78. [PubMed: 15695744]

42. McAlinden NM, Oei TP. Validation of the Quality of Life Inventory for patients with anxiety and depression. Compr Psychiatry. 2006; 47(4):307–14. [PubMed: 16769306]

43. Erbes CR, Kaler ME, Schult T, Polusny MA, Arbisi PA. Mental health diagnosis and occupational functioning in National Guard/Reserve veterans returning from Iraq. J Rehabil Res Dev. 2011; 48(10):1159–70. [PubMed: 22234661]

44. VA National Center for PTSD. [accessed May 5, 2012] Using the PTSD Checklist (PCL). Available at http://www.ptsd.va.gov/professional/pages/assessments/ptsd-checklist.asp

45. Bliese PD, Wright KM, Adler AB, Cabrera O, Castrol CA, Hoge CW. Validating the primary care posttraumatic stress disorder screen and the posttraumatic stress disorder checklist with soldiers returning from combat. J Consult Clin Psychol. 2008; 76:272–81. [PubMed: 18377123]

46. Walker EA, Newman E, Dobie DJ, Cicchanowski P, Katon W. Validation of the PTSD Checklist in an HMO sample of women. Gen Hosp Psychiatry. 2002; 24(6):375–80. [PubMed: 12490338]

47. Sherman JJ, Carlson CR, Wilson JF, Okeson JP, McCubbin JA. Post-traumatic stress disorder among patients with orofacial pain. J Orofac Pain. 2005; 19(4):309–17. [PubMed: 16279482]

48. Litz BT, Stein N, Delancy E, et al. Moral injury and moral repair in war veterans: a preliminary model and intervention strategy. Clin Psychol Rev. 2009; 29(8):695–706. [PubMed: 19683376]

78

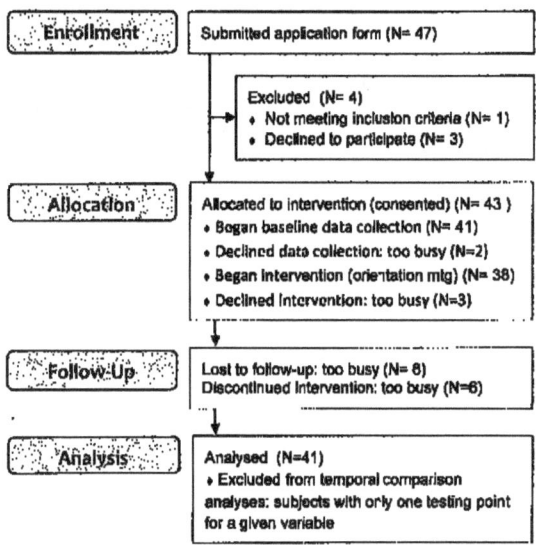

FIGURE 1.
Subjects flow diagram (*N* refers to dyads).

TABLE I

Demographics

	Veteran	Partner
Age (Years)		
Mean	34	29.3
Median	36	31.5
SD	6.7	6.9
Sex (N)		
Male	38	4
Female	5	39
Ethnicity (N)		
White	37	37
Black	1	2
Hispanic/Latin	2	3
Native American	3	1
Education (N)		
Some High School	1	0
High School Graduate	15	9
Some College	14	18
Technical School	1	3
BA	13	12
MA	1	1

Collinge et al.

TABLE II

Weekly Frequency and Duration of Project Activities ($N = 43$ Dyads)

Activity	Veterans (168 Reports)		Partners (176 Reports)	
	Frequency Mean (SD)	Minutes[a] Mean (SD)	Frequency Mean (SD)	Minutes[a] Mean (SD)
Centering Exercise	1.2 (1.9)	9.0 (3.1)	1.4 (1.9)	8.8 (2.3)
Connecting Exercise	0.7 (1.0)	9.3 (3.4)	0.8 (1.1)	8.9 (2.7)
Deep Relaxation Exercise	1.3 (1.7)	12.8 (5.5)	1.1 (1.7)	12.5 (5.1)
Movement Into Stillness	0.5 (1.0)	9.1 (3.4)	0.6 (0.9)	8.7 (2.0)
Sound Into Silence	0.5 (1.1)	9.5 (3.1)	0.5 (1.0)	8.7 (2.1)
Therapeutic Yawning	2.2 (2.8)	8.2 (1.6)	1.9 (2.6)	8.5 (2.2)
Cumulative Mind/Body	6.3 (5.7)	27.0 (17.6)	6.3 (5.6)	27.6 (15.6)
Used Any of the CD	1.5 (2.0)	11.9 (5.8)	1.9 (2.4)	10.4 (4.7)
Watched Any of the DVD	0.6 (1.3)	12.5 (5.7)	0.6 (1.2)	12.4 (6.4)
Looked at the Manual	0.6 (1.2)	9.7 (3.9)	0.9 (1.4)	8.8 (2.8)
Gave Massage	1.3 (1.5)	15.6 (6.6)	1.4 (1.3)	19.4 (6.1)
Received Massage	1.5 (1.6)	18.4 (5.9)	1.1 (1.3)	16.3 (6.5)
Cumulative of All Activities	11.9 (9.2)	66.0 (38.1)	12.2 (8.8)	67.9 (31.6)

[a] For sessions performed, cumulative is total minutes reported per subject.

TABLE III

Symptom Ratings Pre- and Postmassage (Veterans)[a] (Wilcoxon Signed-Rank Tests)

Symptom	Before	After	N	S	P
	Mean (SD)	Mean (SD)			
Physical Pain	3.35 (2.11)	2.36 (1.46)	211	3933.5	<0.001
Physical Tension	4.12 (2.09)	2.30 (1.37)	212	8382.5	<0.001
On Edge/Irritable	3.97 (2.22)	2.06 (1.21)	212	8,055	<0.001
Anxiety/Worry	3.63 (2.21)	2.12 (1.30)	206	5,975	<0.001
Depression	2.59 (2.06)	1.77 (1.24)	212	2332.5	<0.001
Other	1.65 (2.01)	1.34 (1.11)	119	28	<0.010

[a] Self-ratings from 0 (not at all) to 10 (worst imaginable).

TABLE IV

Change in Premassage Symptom Ratings Over Time: Kendall's tau-b Results ($N = 215$ Session Reports)

Symptom	t	p
Physical Pain	−0.023	<0.665
Physical Tension	−0.124	<0.017
On Edge/Irritable	−0.111	<0.032
Anxiety/Worry	−0.048	<0.359
Depression	−0.029	<0.587
Other	−0.043	<0.536

TABLE V

Survey Data: Baseline vs. 4-Week and 8-Week Follow-Up (N=41 Veterans, N=41 Partners, Wilcoxon Signed-Rank Tests)

Instrument	Subjects	Baseline Mean (SD)	4-Week Follow-Up				8-Week Follow-Up			
			Mean (SD)	Percentage Improved (%)	S	p	Mean (SD)	Percentage Improved (%)	S	p
PCL-C	Veterans	34.7 (13.6)	29.0 (9.6)	72.4	106.5	<0.003	29.8 (12.5)	73.3	139.5	<0.003
	Partners	31.8 (11.1)	27.5 (8.4)	59.3	81	<0.026	27.1 (10.8)	67.7	111.5	<0.009
PSS-10	Veterans	26.5 (6.8)	24.6 (6.8)	62.1	59	<0.201	25.2 (7.0)	60	83	<0.088
	Partners	26.7 (6.6)	23.2 (6.3)	66.7	97.5	<0.006	23.6 (6.9)	58.1	103	<0.016
BDI-II	Veterans	12.6 (11.5)	9.0 (7.7)	69	113	<0.008	9.6 (9.0)	66.7	129	<0.006
	Partners	10.1 (7.8)	6.3 (7.2)	66.7	88	<0.015	7.5 (9.4)	67.7	88	<0.032
Compassionate Love Scale	Veterans	83.5 (12.1)	88.1 (14.5)	72.4	58.5	<0.212	84.1 (14.4)	66.7	-35.5	<0.453
	Partners	91.1 (10.6)	91.4 (12.5)	77.8	-25	<0.513	87.2 (15.6)	64.5	-58	<0.216
Self-compassion Scale	Veterans	3.0 (0.6)	3.4 (0.7)	75.9	130.5	<0.003	3.2 (0.9)	70	84	<0.069
	Partners	3.0 (0.8)	3.3 (0.7)	63	100.5	<0.013	3.2 (0.7)	67.7	92	<0.057

84

MEDICAL ACUPUNCTURE
Volume 23, Number 4, 2011
© Mary Ann Liebert, Inc.
DOI: 10.1089/acu.2011.0840

Acupuncture for the Trauma Spectrum Response: Scientific Foundations, Challenges to Implementation

Wayne B. Jonas, MD,[1] Joan A.G. Walter, JD, PA,[1] Matt Fritts, MPH,[1] and Richard C. Niemtzow, MD, PhD, MPH, Col (Ret), USAF, MC, FS[2,*]

ABSTRACT

The long wars in Iraq and Afghanistan have produced extensive and often repeated trauma to United States service members and their families. These injuries occur to the mind, the brain, the body and the soul. The current approach to management of these injuries follows the standard medical model that attempts to isolate the pathophysiological locations and processes affected by the injury and provide specialized care for that part of the person—psychological treatment for mind injuries, neurological treatment for brain injuries, and surgical and rehabilitation approaches for body injuries. This model is overwhelmingly dominated by the use of drugs for symptom management. Yet, research has shown that, no matter where an injury is located, its impact and the healing responses to it cut across these boundaries resulting in a common symptomatic and functional spectrum. The authors of this article have called this the war-related trauma spectrum response (wrTSR) and propose a better approach to this spectrum, which is to induce whole-person healing responses not specialized to addressing the injury cause or location. Acupuncture appears to be such an approach. This article reviews the conceptual and scientific foundations of wrTSR, makes the case for managing it in a holistic manner, and reviews the evidence for using acupuncture as a treatment across the trauma response spectrum. This article then discusses the challenges to implementing of acupuncture in the military and veterans' systems and proposes direct comparative effectiveness, health services, and program evaluation approaches to providing the evidence needed to broaden acupuncture's use.

Key Words: Acupuncture, Military, Pain, Trauma Spectrum Response, TBI, PTSD, Depression, Anxiety, Moral Injury, Integrative Medicine

INTRODUCTION

THE CURRENT WARS in Iraq (Operation Iraqi Freedom, OIF) and Afghanistan (Operation Enduring Freedom, OEF) are returning thousands of warfighters with psychological mind injuries, such as post-traumatic stress disorder (PTSD), and physical mind–body injuries such as traumatic brain injury (TBI), many with long-term symptomatic and functional consequences.[1,2] The multicomponent and overlapping nature of injuries in returning warfighters are appropriately considered as war-related, trauma spectrum responses (wrTSR) and may be of a different character and require a different approach than the civilian trauma stress response (TSR). Trauma to the head and neck occurs in 15%–20% of all battle injuries, and mild TBI (mTBI) may afflict up to 28% of all deployed warfighters.[3,4]

[1]Samueli Institute, Alexandria VA.
[2]United States Air Force Acupuncture Center, Joint Base Andrews MD.

*The opinions and assertions contained herein are the private views of the author and are not to be construed as official or as reflecting the views of the United States Air Force Medical Corps, the Air Force at large, or the Department of Defense. The author indicates that he does not have any conflicts of interest.

249

250   JONAS ET AL.

More than 46% of blast patients and 55% of amputees at Walter Reed Army Medical Center (WRAMC) have sustained comorbid brain injuries. Nearly 20% of soldiers returning from the wars in Iraq and Afghanistan suffer from diagnosable post-traumatic stress disorder (PTSD),[5,6] and nearly 40% report stress-related symptoms and dysfunctions that significantly prevent reintegration into a full, productive life. As stated by Potash, the wounded veteran presents the health care system with "new challenges" not the least of which is the "growing number of patients with co-morbid chronic pain...brain trauma and...attendant cognitive issues."[7]

Triggered by combined mind-brain/body injuries (MBIs), the various manifestations of wrTSR share many common pathophysiological and recovery mechanisms. Evidence supports the potential for the development, expression and durability of certain types of pain and psychopathologies in which genotypic factors could be either latent or code for phenotypes (e.g., of ion channels, neurotransmitters, receptors and synaptic elements) that are differentially expressed from factors from the internal and external environments. In such genotypically predisposed individuals, environmental and/or psychosocial insult can induce a core constellation of common symptoms that includes: (1) psychological and emotional distress (e.g., depression, anxiety, or anger); (2) cognitive impairment; (3) chronic and, often refractory, pain of organic and psychosomatic origins; (4) drug/opioid desensitization (with abuse potential); and (5) somatic (sleep, appetite, sexual, and energy) dysfunction.

Best estimates suggest that multiple comorbidities after exposure to trauma may be present in a substantial percent of wounded military personnel. Villano et al.,[8] and Shipherd and coworkers[9] have shown that psychiatric conditions, such as depression and anxiety, appear to be responsible for the co-occurrence of a syndrome of chronic pain and heightened stress-reactivity, including frank presentation of PTSD, in between 24% and 66% of combat-wounded veterans of OIF/OEF. The impairment of cognitive abilities in patients with chronic pain and PTSD, and the reported incidence and prevalence of chronic pain, PTSD, other neuropsychiatric conditions, and cognitive deficits in wounded OIF/OEF troops has also been described by Beck and colleagues.[10,11] These results are strengthened by the report that more than 60% of these soldiers have been diagnosed with some form of brain-injury condition or apparent constellation of cognitive, emotional, and behavioral features resulting from neural insult.[9] When induced by exposure to deployment and battle, we refer to this constellation of trauma-related manifestations as wrTSRs (Fig. 1).

The current authors hypothesize that the effects of mind-brain injury are approached better by assessing the full spectrum of trauma-related morbidities—rather than dividing them into subcomponents—and then treating the whole person with an approach that enhances the patient's inherent

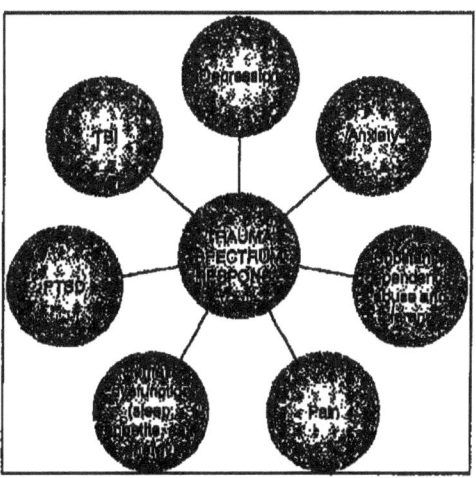

FIG. 1.   Trauma spectrum response components. TBI, traumatic brain injury, PTSD, post-traumatic stress disorder.

healing mechanisms and capacities.[12] The current authors hypothesize that this can be done with a standardized acupuncture method. Using this approach, the authors will test the efficacy of acupuncture on Health Related Quality of Life (HRQoL) and wrTSR comorbidities in service members with TBI and PTSD drawn from several Department of Defense (DoD) and Veterans Affairs (VA) sites across the country.

PTSD AND wrTSR

PTSD as a Component of wrTSR

PTSD (from psychological or mind injuries) is a widely recognized consequence of combat trauma and frequently accompanies wrTBI and bodily injury. The PTSD prevalence rate in OIF/OEF active duty, deployed service members is estimated to be between 15.6% and 17.1%.[13] A more-recent study by the RAND Corporation put this rate at nearly 20%.[6,14] Likewise, the National Vietnam Veterans Readjustment Study (NVVRS[15]) found that more than 15% of male Vietnam theater veterans (VTVs) met criteria for current PTSD, and 30% met diagnostic criteria for lifetime PTSD, while 9% of female VTVs met current PTSD criteria and 27% met lifetime criteria for PTSD related to Vietnam combat trauma. High rates of PTSD and depression (ranging from 9% to 31%, depending on the level of functional impairment reported) are accompanied in nearly half the cases by alcohol abuse or aggressive behavior comorbidity.[14] According to the official report of the Joint Mental Health Advisory Team 7 (J-MHAT 7),

2010 prevalence rates of acute stress, depression and anxiety among deployed OIF/OEF service members are 17.4%, 7.9%, and 8.8%, respectively.[16]

PTSD (especially combat-related PTSD) commonly co-occurs with other psychiatric disorders. In fact, the majority of individuals with PTSD meet criteria for at least one other psychiatric disorder and many for three or more[17,18] including: depression,[19,20] suicide,[21–23] substance abuse disorders,[13,24] anxiety disorders,[18] and chronic pain.[25–28] Comorbid diagnoses are particularly common among people suffering from combat-related PTSD with many in more than 50%.[29,30] Any additional disorders in the presence of PTSD complicates the treatment process and weakens the prognosis for recovery.[17,31,32]

Injury and Trauma to the Soul

In combat, perpetrating, failing to prevent, or witnessing acts that transgress deeply held values can shatter an individual's beliefs about the purpose and meaning of life, challenge belief in God, induce moral conflict, and even precipitate an existential crisis.[34] In December 2009, Veteran's Administration mental health professionals described a new concept of the consequences of spiritual and psychological trauma: "moral injury," defined as "perpetrating, failing to prevent, or bearing witness to acts that transgress deeply held moral beliefs and expectations."[35] Clinicians have observed that moral injury is a significant contributor to clinical depression, addiction, violent behavior, and suicide, and that the current wars create conditions that increase the exposure to moral injury.[36] Signs and symptoms of moral injury include misconduct, violence, other disciplinary problems, social alienation, alienation from self, loss of faith, and loss of meaning.[37]

Prevalence rates for moral injury are not yet available, because it is a relatively new construct, and a well-validated metric is lacking. (A 14-item Moral Injury Scale [MI Scale] has been developed as part of the Marine Resiliency Study [MRS][38] but this scale has not yet been validated in the military.) However, surrogate statistics can be used to estimate the magnitude of the problem. The 2010 MHAT-VII survey found that <15% of soldiers report high or very high individual morale, and 13% report suicidal ideation. Suicide rates among active duty military and veterans are currently alarmingly high and rising.[39] Suicide rates have doubled among Marines in the last 3 years, and these rates remain more than double the national average among Army personnel.

PTSD and Substance Abuse

Substance-use disorders (including alcohol and drug abuse, and dependence) represent another class of disorders commonly co-occurring with PTSD. In two community studies of Vietnam veterans with PTSD, 22%[33] and 39%[24] also had current alcohol abuse or dependence. One hy-

pothesis for this phenomenon is that people with PTSD use alcohol and drugs as a means of self-medicating to relieve their debilitating symptoms.[18] This hypothesis is supported by the finding that a diagnosis of PTSD increases a person's risk of developing an alcohol and drug use disorder. However, research has also demonstrated that people with PTSD (particularly males) are more likely than others with a similar background to have an alcohol use disorder that preceded PTSD.[40,41]

Whatever the cause of comorbidity between PTSD and alcohol/drug use disorders, it is clear that excessive use can worsen the symptoms related to PTSD, including sleep disturbance, difficulty in concentrating, emotional numbing, social isolation, anger and irritability, depression, and hypervigilance. Alcohol can also reduce a person's ability to cope with traumatic memories and stress. A number of factors complicate the treatment of comorbid PTSD and alcohol-use disorder. While, to a patient, alcohol use may appear to help symptoms of PTSD by decreasing the severity and number of nightmares, alcohol may also exacerbate the cycle of avoidance that occurs in PTSD.[42] Furthermore, people with comorbid PTSD and alcohol abuse/dependence are at increased risk for premature termination of therapy, and take a longer time to remit from an episode of chronic PTSD.[31,32]

PTSD and Pain

A number of studies have been conducted to assess the co-occurrence of PTSD and chronic pain symptoms. Benedikt and Kolb reported that 10% of 225 patients referred to a VA pain clinic met criteria for PTSD.[25] Muse reported that 9.5% of a sample of patients attending a multidisciplinary chronic pain center met criteria for "posttraumatic pain syndrome."[43] Patients referred for assessments of chronic pain resulting from a traumatic event have an even higher prevalence of PTSD. In a study conducted to determine the extent to which work-related injuries were associated with PTSD, assessments of 139 injured workers with chronic pain referred to a rehabilitation program indicated that 34.7% reported symptoms consistent with PTSD.[44] Rates of PTSD in patients for which pain is secondary to a motor vehicle accident range from 30% to 50%.[45–47] Geisser et al. examined self-reports of pain, affective distress, and disability in pain patients with and without PTSD symptoms.[48] The results of this study indicated that patients with accident-related pain and high PTSD symptoms reported higher levels of pain and affective distress, compared to patients with accident-related pain who did not have PTSD.

Studies examining the prevalence of chronic pain in patients with a primary diagnosis of PTSD have reported even higher rates of other comorbid conditions. McFarlane et al. reported that pain was the most common physical complaint (45% back pain and 34% headaches) in a sample of PTSD patients reporting physical symptoms.[26] Beckham et al.

performed a study to investigate chronic pain patterns in Vietnam veterans with PTSD[27] and found that 80% reported the presence of a chronic pain condition. In addition, increased levels of PTSD involving reexperiencing of symptoms were associated with increased pain levels and pain-related disability. White and Faustman reported that 60% of 543 veterans treated for PTSD had an identified medical problem and that 1 in 4 had signs some type of musculoskeletal or pain problem.[28]

The co-occurrence of pain and PTSD may have implications for both conditions. Patients with chronic pain related to trauma and PTSD experience more intense pain and affective distress,[48,49] higher levels of life interference,[50] and greater disability than pain patients without trauma or PTSD.[51] Chibnal and Duckro found that patients with PTSD and traumatic headache pain had higher levels of depression and suppressed anger than non-PTSD traumatic headache pain patients.[46] In addition, patients with post-traumatic headache reported more frequent pain and had a poorer prognosis than did nontraumatic headache patients.[52] Thus, the presence of both PTSD and chronic pain may increase the symptom severity of either condition. In the proposed

study, acupuncture treatment in combat-injured soldiers is intended to improve recovery from both conditions and interrupt the trajectory of chronic PTSD and pain symptoms.

Traumatic Brain Injury and wrTSR

TBI is a major cause of death and disability in young people, involving more than 5 million Americans and an annual cost of nearly $50 billion.[53-55] More than 7000 noncombat patients are admitted to VA and military hospitals for TBI annually, with an additional 1700 resulting from problems related to the recent wars in Iraq and Afghanistan.[3,4] Approximately 28% of service members (SMs) with battle injuries requiring evacuation to WRAMC have had TBI.[4] Trauma to the head and neck occurs in 15%–20% of all SMs with battle injuries and mild TBI (mTBI) may afflict up to 28% of all deployed warfighters.[3,4] More than 46% of blast patients and 55% of amputees at WRAMC have sustained comorbid brain injuries.[56,57]

Symptoms and dysfunction, from mild-to-moderate TBI cross the spectrum of dimensions in wrTSR and may include physical symptoms (headache, dizziness, balance, visual

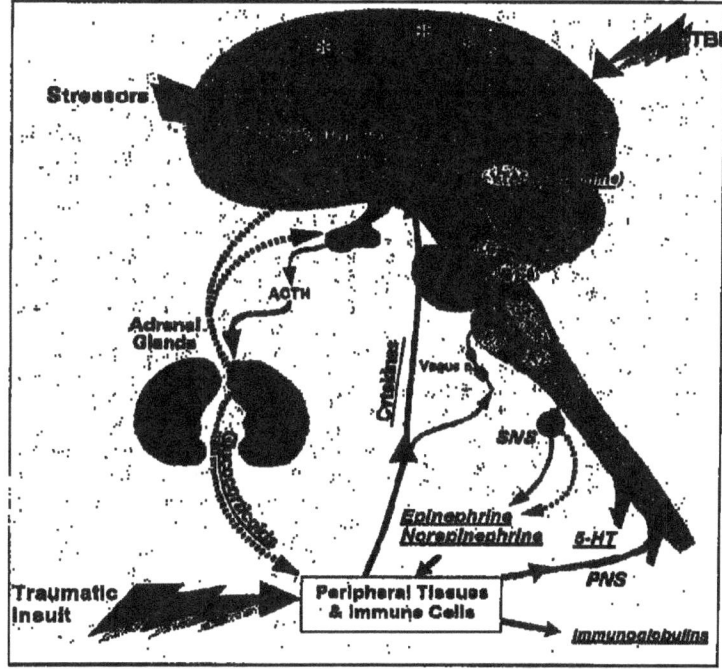

FIG. 2 The hypothalamic–pituitary–adrenal (HPA) axis. Dotted lines represent negative regulatory pathways, solid lines represent positive regulatory pathways. Reprinted with permission from *Annual Review of Immunology*, Volume 20, 2002 by Annual Reviews (www.annualreviews.org). TBI, traumatic brain injury; CRH, corticotrophin releasing hormone; AVN, arginine vasopressin; ACTH, adrenocorticotrophin hormone; SNS, sympathetic nervous system; PNS, parasympathetic nervous system.

changes, and pain), cognitive dysfunction (memory, atten tion, and concentration difficulties), and psychological or behavioral problems (depression, anxiety, anger, mood swings, social and family dysfunctions).[58] Patients admitted to the hospital for other injuries may have sustained previously unrecognized brain injuries or suffer from psychological and stress traumas. The mechanisms and manifestations of TBI from combat blast injuries may have different and more complex characteristics than civilian blunt head injuries.

Wounded military personnel also have unique demographic factors that cause trauma-related physical and psychological injuries to manifest in a particular way. First, this patient population may be comprised of young(er) individuals with characteristically multiple, compound traumas that involve substantial alterations in physical and mental status, and which require acute, subacute, and long-term therapeutic support in both curative and palliative domains.[59] Second, the personal protective equipment that is currently used by the military has undergone significant improvement over its iterations in previous wars. But while such gear has proven to reduce combat-related mortality, the enhanced survival afforded by Kevlar head and torso equipment has led to an increased morbidity of IED-induced injuries, including blast-generated appendicular fractures, projectile wounds, traumatic amputation(s), and compression wounds as well as concussive (and cerebral contusive) insults.[4]

Finally, such external-blast TBI (ebTBI) is more often accompanied by skull fractures, seizures, and limb amputations. (For a summary, please see Warden and French 2005 and Warden 2006.[3,4]) Rates of post-concussive symptoms (PCS) may occur at increased frequency than found in civilian populations.[4] MTBIs sustained in battle may be difficult to distinguish from, and are often accompanied by, PTSD. Thus, both MTBI and PTSD often manifest with similar sets of symptoms and dysfunctions.[60]

Converging Mechanisms of wrTSR

As illustrated in Figure 2, there are interactive peripheral and central mechanisms that affect the progression of the constellation of features representative of wrTSR. Both physical insult to peripheral tissues and the concomitant stress that such an injury evokes induce this cascade of events to produce early and late effects across the trauma spectrum. These interacting mechanisms produce high levels of inflammatory mediators, including the cytokines (most notably interleukins [IL]–1 and – 6), tumor necrosis factor-alpha (TNF-α), neurotropic factors and the tachykinins (including substance P).[61] These "bottom-up" mediators can affect the central nervous system (CNS), both by engagement of the peripheral nervous system and by accessing the CNS via altering the vascular integrity and permeability of the brain, to evoke neuroinflammatory changes within the brain parenchyma. The cytokines and tachykinins affect glial metabolism and disrupt glial–neuronal calcium

regulation, leading to increased neural uptake and endocellular release of calcium.

Acting as an intracellular messenger, calcium produces "downstream" effects to induce early and late-stage transcriptional factors and promotes translation of ion channel, synaptic, enzymatic, and receptor proteins that can lead to disrupted neural function in several brain areas (for a summary see Carofoli and Klee, 1999).[62] This aberrant neural and glial activity is manifested in alteration of both neurochemistry (of neurotransmitter and metabolic systems; for example, epinephrine, norepinephrine, serotonin [5-hydroxytryptamine; 5-HT], and dopamine, as well as other peptidergic and amino-acid transmitters) and of more global network properties to produce "top-down" brain-mind effects that induce pathological change(s) in mentation, cognition, and psychological states (see Fig. 2). Thus, while initial effects may be transitory, more durable sequelae are evidenced in those systems with the highest "vulnerability," namely, those neural networks and systems that have sustained direct neurological damage and those with genotic-phenotypic predispositions. These factors are strong predictors of the development of chronic pain, pain syndromes, and psychopathology following trauma.[63]

Some of these effects are overt and acute, while others are more subtle and delayed, reflecting the slower changes that occur as a central consequence of inflammatory processes, with resultant alterations in neural and glial function, and disruption and/or remodeling of neurological networks. The lack of explicit, first-order signs and symptoms may result in a return to combatant status, or, if other wounds are sufficiently grave, triage to a secondary- or tertiary-care facility. Often, it is in these settings—or in the home—that the signs and symptoms reflective of progression along the pain and neuropsychopathologic spectrum of wrTSR (i.e., co-occurrence of depression and anxiety—including PTSD—disorders) are more saliently expressed and and in evidence. This is not incidental; rather, it may at least partially be the result of the psychophysiological effects of increased allostatic loads incurred by social, familial, occupational, and/or economic stressors.[64] The reciprocity and cyclicity of these events are such that:

1. Large-scale peripheral injury augments the inflammatory effects within the CNS.
2. Geno- and phenotypic factors are induced/provoked that are ultimately expressed as pain and psychopathology.
3. These pathologies become chronic, with possible functional and structural remodeling of CNS micro-networks
4. These networks mediate dysfunctional responses and reactions to environmental factors.
5. This adaptational dissonance enhances stress loads.
6. The condition(s) may worsen as discordant interactions between the underlying neural state and environmental factors become increasingly synergistic (Fig. 2).[12,65]

While symptomatic assessment is important, if not essential, to diagnose syndrome expression accurately within this spectrum disorder, and, ultimately, to determine the best type(s) of care, it is equally important to attempt to identify peripheral and central biological markers (e.g., IL 1 and 6, immunoglobulin G, cortisol) and endproduct metabolites of adrenergic (i.e., 3-methoxy, 4-hydroxy phenylglycol [MHPG]), dopaminergic (i.e., homovanillic acid [HVA, dihydroxyphenylacetic acid [DOPAC]), and serotonergic (i.e., 5-hydroxyindole acetic acid [5-HIAA]) neurotransmission (see below, also Fig. 2) that reflect particular syndromes or subsyndromes of the TSR continuum, and physiologic effects of both pathological variables and those of various treatments.

This pathological progression advances many patients to treatment failure, symptomatic worsening, chronic illness, psychosocial stress, and family and life disruption. As described below, there is good evidence to believe some integrative medicine approaches, especially acupuncture, can disrupt this pathological progression and offer an opportunity to reverse this cycle and lead to enhanced recovery, quality of life and function.

PTSD, wrTSR, RESEARCH, AND THE HEALTH CARE SYSTEM

Failure to Address the Full wrTSR and the Overuse and Underuse Burdens on Health Care

The expression of wrTSR complex often manifests following treatment of the acute neuropsychological symptoms caused by in-theater trauma, with signs and symptoms reflective of progression along this neuropsychopathological spectrum in these wounded military personnel.[61] This pathological progression may be the result of psychophysiological effects of increased allostatic loads incurred by social, familial, occupational, and/or economic stressors, and it advances many patients down the slippery slope of treatment failure, symptomatic worsening, psychosocial stress, and life disruption.[62]

These patients are classified into categories based on mind, brain, or bodily damage and sent to specialty clinics (psychiatry, neurology, rehabilitation medicine, etc.) that address selected components of the wrTSR (psychological, neurological, or physical). Often, these SMs simply do not show up for care (avoiding treatment altogether for symptoms that carry a social stigma) or show up repeatedly at a later time in primary care clinics with a variety of somatic complaints involving dysfunctions in sleep, appetite, energy, and/or sexual activity. The former results in under-diagnosis and treatment, and the latter increases the burden on primary care resulting from chronic, unremitting illness. The latter may arise from so-called "subthreshold" PTSD or "mild-to-moderate" TBI, which often goes undiagnosed

or is treated ineffectively.[63] These patients present weeks to months after trauma exposure with symptoms and dysfunctions that chronically burden the DoD or VA health care delivery systems.[7,63] Clearly, the zero-sum nature of this situation is opprobrious to the sound practice of medicine—both technically and ethically—and calls for a more innovative and comprehensive approach to addressing the full consequences of mind–brain/body injuries (MBI).

The Need to Focus Research on the Whole Person wrTSR Response

Clearly, these epidemiological and mechanistic data indicate a large and growing clinical problem (with recent estimates of this pattern of comorbidity within this population of wounded at as much as $n = 10,000$)[66] and suggest that these patterns of comorbidity may reflect underlying, common patho-etiologic variables and mechanisms; compel the need for additional research to define these variables and mechanisms more fully; and equally compel and sustain the need for "the development of intervention based on a new integrated care model."[9] In addition, the long-term impact of MBI goes far beyond individuals and affects their families and communities, which, too often, go unaddressed by the health care system.[67] Thus, from the perspectives of the person, family, and community, there is good reason to consider the full wrTSR (rather than individual components) and to investigate integrative, multidimensional (mind, body, symptom, function) approaches to classification and treatment.

Because of this complex nature of the trauma response, the current standards of care for wrTSR are probably not maximally effective, nor do they address fully the biopsychosocial aspects and spectrum effects of wrTSR. Thus, there is a need for additional research to define and understand TSR more completely so as to develop interventions based upon both neuroscientific information and new integrated care models. Such care should address the whole-person experience of wrTSR and seek to facilitate prevention, cure, and healing as an integrated paradigm that includes contextual understanding of patient-specific variables, uses innovative therapeutic approaches based on rigorous methods of empirical evaluation, and narrows the gap between research and clinical practice.[8] Complementary and integrative approaches, and acupuncture in particular, may be able to address many of these challenges to wrTSR treatment.

Complementary and Integrative Practices

Complementary and integrative medicine (CIM) refers to a family of holistic practices used in conjunction with conventional medicine to enhance health, stimulate recovery, and reduce side-effects. CIM therapies are being increasingly utilized within comprehensive care models[68] and may provide major contributions to patient recovery. Local surveys in military treatment facilities have shown that more than 70% of DoD beneficiaries may use CIM at certain sites.[69] A large survey conducted by the Samueli Institute (Alexandria, VA) in conjunction with the DoD Health Behaviors Survey showed that more than 45% of active duty military members have used CIM and more than two thirds used dietary and nutritional supplements in a 12-month period. Surveys, such as the Klemm Analysis Group[70] and Healthcare Analysis and Information Group[71] reports, showed extensive use of CIM practices by Veterans Health Administration (VHA) health care practitioners.[62] The wide acceptance of CIM for addressing various health issues suggests that, were a CIM approach to prove effective for treating PTSD, many people who have mixed feelings about psychiatric treatment might use CIM.[73] Current research is shifting its primary focus from managing and mitigation of PTSD to one that also promotes post-traumatic adaptation, development, and resurgence. Ai and Park[74] describe three interrelated trends in mental health research that are based on a broader view of (1) the positive psychology movement, (2) the recognition of the role of spirituality and religion in health and well-being, and (3) stress-related growth.[74] Similarly, research on the use of optimal healing environments for the treatment (and possible prevention) of the negative effects of PTSD is emerging.[75]

For the treatment of wrTSR, CIM approaches fall into two basic categories:

1. Actions people do for themselves that enhance self-care and self-treatment skills, such as mind–body practices[76] (imagery, relaxation response,[77] mindfulness training,[78] and yoga[79]), self-care skills (community self-care practices, diet, and exercise training), device-assisted biofeedback (heart-rate monitoring, breathing, and virtual reality), and diet and supplements for enhancing cognitive/physical fitness and psychological resilience
2. Nondrug and nonpsychiatric approaches used by CIM professionals to complement conventional treatments and facilitate healing, such as acupuncture,[80,81] Reiki, osteopathic manipulation,[82] chiropractic, and integrative medicine team approaches.

RESEARCH ON ACUPUNCTURE FOR PTSD AND wTSR

Preliminary Data for the Effectiveness of Acupuncture for HRQoL and wrTSR Comorbidities

Arguably, the most promising CIM intervention for TSR is acupuncture. Originating in China, acupuncture has been used as a medical treatment modality for more than 2500 years, but only relatively recently has it received attention in the United States. It is based on a concept of health and disease that is very different from conventional Western scientific thinking. Acupuncture theory holds that energy, called Qi, travels along pathways (meridians) within the body. Disease states result from disruption or blockage of proper Qi flow. To influence this energy flow, thin metal acupuncture needles are inserted at specific points along the meridians. The stimulation of those points may also be accomplished by other techniques, such as electrical stimulation, laser, moxibustion, and pressure.[83,84]

Acupuncture is used to treat many conditions. Even as far back as 1998, it was estimated that more than 1 million people in the United States collectively received 10 million acupuncture treatments.[85] Treated disorders included acute and chronic pain of various etiologies, nausea, stress and anxiety states, depression, substance abuse, allergic rhinitis, asthma, gastrointestinal disorders, infectious disease, and brain injury from stroke.[84] Overall studies show that acupuncture helps reduce stress, anxiety, and pain, and is effective for treating depression and insomnia, which are all symptoms with diagnostic groups that are part of the complex of the trauma spectrum.[86–91] The relevant studies are summarized next.

Controlled Clinical Studies of Acupuncture

There is evidence, demonstrated via controlled clinical trials, that acupuncture can be effective for treating many of the specific comorbidities that comprise wrTSR in TBI and PTSD. Recent randomized, controlled, blinded studies support the efficacy of acupuncture for treating pain associated with fibromyalgia, knee arthroscopy, and labor.[92–94] These findings are consistent with many prior investigations showing the amelioration of pain caused by diverse conditions in both humans and animals.[95] Strong evidence also exists for treating postoperative nausea and vomiting with acupuncture, resulting in minimal side-effects.[96] Several clinical trials have demonstrated acupuncture's effectiveness for ameliorating stress and anxiety and for facilitating a mentally relaxed state.[97–106] Studies in healthy volunteers have demonstrated reduction in stress scores and levels of subjective stress achieved by acupuncture,[107,108] while another study showed an increase in vagal tone, with suppression of sympathetic tone in healthy volunteers, suggesting a direct effect on CNS control.[109] Acupressure has reduced anxiety and stress as well as perceived pain of treatment in emergency patients being transported to the hospital via ambulance.[101] Electrical stimulation of acupuncture points has been shown to increase "mental relaxation" in patients with chronic physical disorders,[110] and, in another controlled study of acupuncture, muscle sympathetic nerve activity was reduced in heart failure patients undergoing mental stress testing.[111]

Furthermore, acupuncture is effective for addressing other symptoms that comprise wrTSR, including insomnia[112–115] and somatic and postoperative pain.[95,116–121]

While research results for the effectiveness of acupuncture for treating drug addiction is mixed, there are national standards for using ear acupuncture in drug addiction, with reported effectiveness, and several states mandate a trial of acupuncture for treating drug addiction.[122] Several studies in patients with stroke have found that acupuncture can enhance cognitive and physical functioning in patients with brain damage above and beyond conventional rehabilitation approaches.[123] In a study by Hollifield (the acupuncture trainer and consultant on this project) and colleagues, acupuncture was as effective as cognitive behavioral therapy and markedly more effective than a wait-list control for alleviating symptoms of PTSD in veterans.[124] In addition, large randomized controlled trials of acupuncture for treating various chronic pain conditions have shown acupuncture to be more effective than guideline-based standard therapy.[125,126] Finally, numerous case reports, case series, and observational studies have reported benefits in patients after surgery and head trauma.[126–131]

Acupuncture studies frequently use the Short Form (SF)–36/SF-12 for measurement of HRQoL, which will be the primary outcome measure for this study. Across heterogeneous populations, acupuncture consistently improves SF-36 scores by 5–7 points,[132–135] a change that is considered to be clinically significant.

Acupuncture Research in the Military

Several studies overseen by the primary author of this article have been done on acupuncture use in the military for the comorbidities of trauma response. These include studies on acute pain,[73] chronic and refractory pain,[127] and PTSD.[128] The authors are currently testing a simplified field deployable acupuncture technique to be used for headache called Battlefield Acupuncture (BFA), also known as Auricular Stimulation Procedure (ASP), previously tested for pain.[81] This simple Five Point ear acupuncture technique reduced pain by 23% over controls.[81] The authors of the current article have recently completed two studies at WRAMC using acupuncture. One in the Deployment Health Clinical Center found that acupuncture over 12 weeks was acceptable and effective as an adjunct in OIF/OEF patients being treated for PTSD.[†] A second study done in the rehabilitation clinic examined the effect of scalp acupuncture for treating phantom-limb pain in amputees from the war.[‡] In a pilot study, Niemtzow et al.[130] and Gambel et al.[¶] found acupuncture effective for addressing this otherwise refractory pain condition. A follow-up study is being planned that will parallel and coordinate data collection with this proposed study. The current authors have also conducted a

Rapid Evidence Assessment of the Literature (REAL©; which is also reported in this special issue by York et al., pages 229–236). The REAL was conducted to survey the literature on acupuncture research conducted in the military population and to evaluate the quality of the research available—there is a paucity of published reports in this area and further research is necessary, as acupuncture is becoming more readily chosen for military populations in the field for treating various conditions.

Translation of effective therapies is of prime importance for the military. The current authors are currently evaluating the feasibility of training Air Force physicians in the BFA technique for possible widespread use as a pain treatment modality in military primary care. The current study will use an approach recently shown by Hollifield et al. to be effective for trauma spectrum comorbidities in veterans with PTSD. Hollifield et al. used a semi-standardized acupuncture technique that was carefully developed from Traditional Chinese Medicine and matched to trauma response syndromes. In a randomized controlled trial, this approach was found to be easily teachable, as effective as cognitive behavioral therapy, and markedly more effective than a wait-list control for alleviating symptoms of PTSD in veterans.[124] Hollifield also found that this approach was effective for addressing other trauma comorbidities, including pain, insomnia and quality of life.[§]

Common, Interacting Mechanisms of Acupuncture in wrTSR Conditions

Acupuncture may have such ubiquitous effects because it appears to simultaneously influence several common, interacting mechanisms involved in trauma response and recovery. Acupuncture is known to have effects on the autonomic nervous system and the prefrontal cortex—systems that are involved in the pathophysiology of the emotional, pain, and cognitive dysfunctions of TSR.[136–138] It has been established that acupuncture stimulates the release of endogenous opioids and that analgesic effects are blocked in a dose response manner by naloxone, an opioid antagonist.[95] Cho et al. have demonstrated specifically that the cingulate gyrus and the thalamic areas, activated in the presence of applied pain stimulation, show brain activity that correlates with decreased pain sensation in human subjects.[139] There is evidence that electroacupuncture may affect the pressor response, resulting in decreased oxygen demand in the presence of myocardial ischemia[140] and cardiovascular reactivity and hypertension.[141] Thus, acupuncture appears to cause a broad matrix of CNS responses involving the amygdala, hippocampus, hypothalamus,

†Cooper J, Walter J, Ader D, Niemtzow RC. Outcomes and Cost Assessment of Acupuncture in the Treatment (OCAT) of Pain Patients at Malcolm Grow. Unpublished.

‡Engel C, Benedek D, Armstrong D, Osuch E, et al. Acupuncture for the Treatment of Trauma Survivors. Unpublished.

¶Gambel J, Niemtzow RC, Burns SM, Penhollow T, et al. Acupuncture for Post Amputation Limb Pain. Unpublished.

§Jonas WB and Hollifield M. Personal communication about acupuncture techniques effective for trauma. Washington, DC, 2008.

cerebellum, basal ganglia, anterior cingulate, insula, and other limbic structures, as evidenced by functional magnetic resonance imaging, positron emission tomography, and electroencephalographic studies.[156] Responses by the CNS may be dependent on the type and frequency of acupuncture treatment.[136,142,143] In this proposed study, the authors will use an acupuncture approach previously developed and found to be effective for addressing TSR.[124]

Specific and Nonspecific Effects of Acupuncture

The many potential mechanisms for the efficacy of acupuncture on the trauma recovery spectrum has both pros and cons for testing its efficacy. The apparent "multimechanism" whole-person's response acupuncture seems to provide a compelling rationale for testing acupuncture effects on quality of life and function in two heterogenious populations—the authors expect both to improve significantly. The down side for collecting evidence about acupuncture efficacy is that it becomes difficult to select an appropriate control procedure without knowing its precise mechanism. Three competing mechanisms exist: (1) the traditional Chinese theory of "point specificity"; (2) the more Western explanations related to facia and the induction of facia/neural/inflammatory "matrix" responses; and (3) the "therapeutic meaning and expectancy" theory of acupuncture as a placebo. While all three of these potential mechanisms cannot be disentangled in a single clinical trial, the acupuncture control methods will be specifically selected to control for all three mechanisms simultaneously in the following manner.

Clinical trials testing the therapeutic claims of acupuncture have focused on the efficacy of needling at specific sites on the body surface (acupuncture points), using selected needling techniques. The choices of acupuncture points and needling techniques are guided by traditional and modern theories and diagnostic procedures. However, insertion of needles into the body can also induce a range of physiological effects that are not dependent on the location of stimulation and are thus considered nonspecific.[144,145] Among these nonspecific effects likely to be associated with the microtrauma of acupuncture are stimulation of cutaneous microcirculation,[146,147] heterosegmental analgesic mechanisms (i.e., diffuse noxious inhibitory control),[148,149] and aspects of the relaxation response.[150,151] Even "needle grasp"—a biomechanical phenomenon traditionally associated with acupuncture, needle insertion, and manipulation—has been shown to occur to a marked, albeit lesser, extent at control points relative to acupuncture points.[152] The realization that acupuncture treatment elicits nonspecific and specific effects has led to adoption of the term "sham acupuncture" for control needling procedures in randomized controlled trials (RCTs) of acupuncture, because the term "placebo" is generally applied to control procedures that are believed to be inert.

Nonspecific effects of needling may well have contributed to the outcomes of recent large-scale German trials of acupuncture (involving several hundred to several thousand patients per trial) in which sham acupuncture, delivered as superficial needling at non-acupuncture points with no needle manipulation, was found to be as effective as true acupuncture for treating low-back pain[132,153] and migraine.[135,154] Invasive sham acupuncture cannot be discarded as a control procedure in acupuncture trials, however, in part because another of the German trials, one on osteoarthritis of the knee,[133] found acupuncture to be statistically superior to the same type of "minimal acupuncture" provided in the low-back pain and migraine trials cited above.

The likelihood that invasive needling at non-acupuncture points induces some level of nonspecific healing has led to the development of an alternative type of sham acupuncture involving noninvasive needling.[155,156] This procedure utilizes needles with blunted tips, designed such that contact with the skin leads to retraction into the shaft instead of penetration of the skin. Despite nonpenetration, the sham needle is held "upright" because it perforates the tape used to hold a small O ring in place that surrounds the needle placement site[155] or the sham needle perforates a small square of Styrofoam that is attached at the site of "needling."[156] In either procedure, the patient sees the needle shorten and believes that true acupuncture has occurred—an expectation that has been confirmed by questionnaires. A review of the literature over the period since these nonpenetrating sham needles were introduced in 1999 reveals 19 RCTs that utilized a sham needling telescoping device, of which 8 trials were positive, 9 negative, and 2 mixed with regard to their authors' stated primary outcomes. The summative situation with respect to trial results is similarly inconclusive in acupuncture trials that used invasive needling as a sham control procedure.[157]

At this stage in the development of acupuncture research methodology, it seems clear that an appropriate sham procedure cannot be designed or agreed upon until a clearer understanding emerges regarding the mechanism by which the acupuncture needle elicits its response.[158] Given the present dilemma, the current authors have chosen to utilize a noninvasive needling procedure for a sham control in the present 3-arm trial of acupuncture for HRQoL in TBI and PTSD. This procedure will be designed to control for the "meaning responses" (placebo)[159] associated with the delivery of acupuncture and, when compared to true acupuncture, will allow an assessment of the treatment benefit that results from acupuncture needling-related responses.

CONCLUSIONS

There is a need for new approaches for treatment of trauma that induce a whole-person healing response. The current medical approaches that divide an individual into subspecialties increase the precision of diagnosis and treatment but create complicated management approaches, which are, in some cases, counterproductive. Healing approaches such as acupuncture provide an alternative model to the current biomedical model and provide an opportunity for widespread healing with fewer medications and subspecialty oversight, and are nonstigmatizing.

However, the costs of differing strategies for delivery of acupuncture may vary substantially. Little research has evaluated the cost effectiveness of acupuncture treatment or determined which strategies are optimal for adoption. A recent panel conducted by the RAND–Samueli Program on Integrative Medicine Policy focused on economic analysis issues in CIM, which will help inform the DoD about the best approaches for evaluating these differing strategies. The report and toolkit from that panel should be out before the end of 2011. Given the growing interest in acupuncture and integrative approaches for treating wrTSR, such as that incorporated to the recent DoD Pain Task Force Report, and given the increased suffering likely to emerge as warriors return from the battlefield with the coming drawdown, it would behoove the military and the VA to substantially accelerate the development and evaluation of programs delivering acupuncture. SMs and families who are suffering the consequences of these long wars deserve nothing less than the optimal healing environments we can provide.

ACKNOWLEDGMENTS

The authors would like to thank Cindy Crawford, BA, and Jarrad Davis, BA, for assistance in preparation of the manuscript and Jim Giordano, PhD, for contributions to the concept of wrTSR. This study article was partially funded by a grant from the Department of Defense Telemedicine and Advanced Technology Research Center.

DISCLOSURE STATEMENT

The authors have neither conflicts of interest nor financial disclosures to report.

REFERENCES

1. Erbes C, Westermeyer J, Engdahl B, Johnsen E. Post-traumatic stress disorder and service utilization in a sample of service members from Iraq and Afghanistan. *Mil. Med.* 2007;172(4):359–363.
2. Hoge CW, Auchterlonie JL, Milliken CS. Mental health problems, use of mental health services, and attrition from military service after returning from deployment to Iraq or Afghanistan. *JAMA.* 2006;295(9):1023–1032.
3. Warden DL, French L. Traumatic brain injury in the war zone. *N Engl J Med.* 2005;353(6):633–634.
4. Warden D. Military TBI during the Iraq and Afghanistan wars. *J Head Trauma Rehabil.* 2006;21(5):398–402.
5. Engelhard IM, Huijding J, van den Hout MA, de Jong PJ. Vulnerability associations and symptoms of post-traumatic stress disorder in soldiers deployed to Iraq. *Behav Res Ther.* 2007;45(10):2317–2325.
6. Coulter I, Ellison M, Hilton L, Rhodes H, Ryan G. *Hospital-Based Integrative Medicine: A Case Study of the Barriers and Factors Facilitating the Creation of a Center, vol MG-519-NCCAM.* Santa Monica, CA: RAND Corporation; 2008.
7. Potash M. Chronic pain and co-morbid brain injury from IED trauma. *Pract Pain Manage.* 2007;7(5):12–17.
8. Villano C, Rosenblum A, Magura S. Prevalence and correlate of posttraumatic stress disorder and chronic severe pain in psychiatric outpatients. *J Rehabil Res Dev.* 2007;44(2):167–178.
9. Shipherd JC, Keyes M, Jovanovic T, et al. Veterans seeking treatment for posttraumatic stress disorder: What about comorbid chronic pain? *J Rehabil Res Dev.* 2007;44(2):153–166.
10. Beck J, Gudmundsdottir B, Shipherd J. PTSD and emotional distress symptoms measured after a motor vehicle accident: Relationship with pain coping profiles. *J Psychopathol Behav Assess.* 2003;54(4):219–227.
11. Beck J, Palyo S, Winer E, Schwagler B, Ang E. Virtual reality exposure therapy for PTSD symptoms after a road accident: An uncontrolled case series. *Behav Ther.* 2007;38(1):39–48.
12. Giordano J, Walter J. Pain and psychopathology in military wounded: How etiology, epidemiology sustain an ethics of treatment. *Pract Pain Manage.* 2007;7(6):34–42.
13. Hoge CW, Castro CA, Messer SC, McGurk D, Cotting DI, Koffman RL. Combat duty in Iraq and Afghanistan, mental health problems, and barriers to care. *N Engl J Med.* 2004;351(1):13–22.
14. Tanielian T, Jaycox, L, eds. *Invisible Wounds of War: Psychological and Cognitive Injuries, Their Consequences and Services to Assist Recovery.* Santa Monica, CA: RAND Center for Military Health Policy Research; 2008.
15. Kulka R. *Trauma and the Vietnam War Generation: Report of Findings From the National Vietnam Veterans Readjustment Study.* New York: Brunner/Mazel; 1990.
16. Office of The Surgeon General, United States Army Medical Command; Office of the Command Surgeon HQ, US-CENTCOM; and Office of the Command Surgeon US Forces Afghanistan (USFOR-A). Report of the Joint Mental Health Advisory Team 7 (J-MHAT 7), February 22, 2011. Online document at: www.armymedicine.army.mil/reports/mhat/mhat_vii/J_MHAT_7.pdf Accessed November 20, 2011.
17. Grinage BD. Diagnosis and management of post-traumatic stress disorder. *Am Fam Phys.* 2003;68(12):2401–2408.
18. Brady K, Killeen T, Brewerton T, Lucerini S. Comorbidity of psychiatric disorers and posttraumatic stress disorder. *J Clin Psychiatr.* 2000;61(7):22–32.
19. Berlim M, Perizzolo J, Fleck M. Posttraumatic stress disorder and major depression. *Rev Bras Psiquiatr.* 2003;25(1):51–54.
20. Bleich A, Koslowsky M, Dolev A, Lerer B. Post-traumatic stress disorder and depression: An analysis of comobidity. *Br J Psychiatr.* 1997;170:479–482.
21. Oquendo MA. Friend JM, Halberstam B, et al. Association of comorbid posttraumatic stress disorder and major de-

pression with greater risk for suicidal behavior. *Am J Psychiatr.* 2003;160(3):580–582.

22. Stein DJ, Bandelow B, Hollander E, et al. WCA Recommendations for the long-term treatment of posttraumatic stress disorder. *CNS Spectr.* 2003;8(8[suppl1]):31–39.

23. Shalev AY, Freedman S, Peri T, et al. Prospective study of posttraumatic stress disorder and depression following trauma. *Am J Psychiatr.* 1998;155(5):630–637.

24. Anonymous. Health status of Vietnam veterans: I. Psychological characteristics: The Centers for Disease Control Vietnam Experience Study. *JAMA.* 1988;259:2701–2707.

25. Benedikt RA, Kolb LC. Preliminary findings on chronic pain and posttraumatic stress disorder. *Am J Psychiatr.* 1986; 143(7):908–910.

26. McFarlane AC, Atchison M, Rafalowicz E, Papay P. Physical symptoms in post-traumatic stress disorder. *J Psychosom Res.* 1994;38(7):715–726.

27. Beckham JC, Crawford AL, Feldman ME, Kirby AC, Hertzberg MA, Davidson JR, Moore SD. Chronic posttraumatic stress disorder and chronic pain in Vietnam combat veterans. *J Psychosom Res.* 1997;43(4):379–389.

28. White P, Faustman W. Coexisting physical conditions among inpatients with post-traumatic stress disorder. *Mil Med.* 1989;154(2):66–71.

29. Forbes D, Creamer M, Hawthorne G, Allen N, McHugh T. Comorbidity as a predictor of symptom change after treatment in combat-related posttraumatic stress disorder. *J Nerv Mental Dis.* 2003;191(2):93–99.

30. Kozaric-Kovacic D, Borovecki A. Prevalence of psychotic comorbidity in combat-related post-traumatic stress disorder. *Mil Med.* 2005;170(3):223–226.

31. Zlotnick C, Warshaw M, Shea M, Allsworth J, Pearlstein T, Keller M. Chronicity in posttraumatic stress disorder (PTSD) and predictors of course of comorbid PTSD in patients with anxiety disorders. *J Traumatic Stress.* 1999;12(1):89–100.

32. Riggs DS, Rukstalis M, Volpicelli JR, Kalmanson D, Foa EB. Demographic and social adjustment characteristics of patients with comorbid posttraumatic stress disorder and alcohol dependence: Potential pitfalls to PTSD treatment. *Addict Behav.* 2003;28(9):1717–1730.

33. Kulka RA, Schlenger WE, Fairbank J. *Trauma and the Vietnam War Generation.* New York: Bruner-Mazel; 1990.

34. Hufford D, Fritts M, Rhodes J. Spiritual fitness. *Mil Med.* 2010;175(8[suppl]):73–87.

35. Litz BT, Stein N, Delaney E, Lebowitz L, Nash WP, Silva C, Maguen S. Moral injury and moral repair in war veterans: A preliminary model and intervention strategy. *Clin Psychol Rev.* 2009;29(8):695–706.

36. SoulRepairProject. Exploring Moral Injury and Religious Resources for Moral Repair in War Veterans. March 18–19, 2011; San Diego, CA. Online document at: https://secure .groundspring.org/dn/index.php?aid=3791 Accessed November 20, 2011.

37. Nash W. Moral injury and moral repair: Overview of constructs and early data [presentation]. Force Health Protection Conference, Phoenix, AZ, August 8–14, 2010.

38. Baker D, et al. Marine Resiliency Study (MRS): Prospective, longitudinal assessment of risk and protective factors for stress injuries and illnesses in ground combat marines [presentation].

Navy and Marine Corps Combat and Operational Stress Conference, San Diego, CA, Washington, DC: D.D; May 18–20, 2010.

39. Marines. Department of Defense Suicide Event Report, Date Signed 2/28/2008, Online document at: www.marines.mil/ news/messages/Pages/MESSAGES140.aspx Accessed November 20, 2011.

40. Davidson J, Kudler H, Saunders W, Smith R. Symptom and comorbidity patterns in world war II and Vietnam veterans with *Posttraumatic Stress Disorder. Comprehensive Psychiatr.* 1990;31:162–170.

41. Sonne SC, Back SE, Diaz Zuniga C, Randall CL, Brady KT. Gender differences in individuals with comorbid alcohol dependence and post-traumatic stress disorder. *Am J Addict.* 2003;12(5):412–423.

42. Kofoed L, Friedman MJ, Peck R. Alcoholism and drug abuse in patients with PTSD. *Psychiatr Q.* 1993;64(2):151–171.

43. Muse M. Stress-related, posttraumatic chronic pain syndrome: Behavioral treatment approach. *Pain.* 1986;25(3):389–394.

44. Asmundson GJ, Norton GR, Allerdings MD, Norton PJ, Larsen DK. Posttraumatic stress disorder and work-related injury. *J Anxiety Disord.* 1998;12(1):57–69.

45. Devini T, Blanchard EB, Hickling EJ, Buckley TC. Effect of psychological treatment on cognitive bias in motor vehicle accident–related post-traumatic stress disorder. *J Anxiety Disord* 2009;18(2):211–231.

46. Chibnall JT, Duckro PN. Post-traumatic stress disorder in chronic post-traumatic headache patients. *Headache.* 1994(34):357–361.

47. Taylor S, Koch WJ. Anxiety disorders due to motor vehicle accidents: Nature and treatment. *Clin Psychol Rev.* 1995(15):721–738.

48. Geisser ME, Roth RS, Bachman JE, Eckert TA. The relationship between symptoms of post-traumatic stress disorder and pain, affective disturbance and disability among patients with accident and non-accident related pain. *Pain.* 1996;66(2–3):207–214.

49. Toomey TC, Seville JL, Abashian SW, Finkel AG, Mann JD. Circumstances of chronic pain onset: Relationship to pain description, coping and psychological distress [abstr]. American Pain Society, Miami Beach, FL; 1994: A–76.

50. Turk DC, Okifuji A, Starz TW, Sinclair JD. Effects of type of symptom onset on psychological distress and disability in fibromyalgia syndrome patients. *Pain.* 1996;68(2–3):423–430.

51. Shennan JJ, Turk DC, Okifuji A. Prevalence and impact of posttraumatic stress disorder-like symptoms on patients with fibromyalgia syndrome. *Clin J Pain.* 2000;16(2):127–134.

52. Tashima WT, Stoddard VM. Ethnic group similarities in the biofeedback treatment of pain. *Med. Psychother.* 1990(3):69–75.

53. Langlois J. *Traumatic Brain Injury in the United States: Assessing Outcomes in Children.* Atlanta, GA: National Center for Injury Prevention and Control of the Centers for Disease Control and Prevention; 2001.

54. Lewin J, Sumners D. Anorexia due to brain injury. *Brain Inj.* 1992;6(2):199–201.

55. Traumatic brain injury among members of active components, US Armed Forces, 1997–2006. Medical Surveillance Monthly Report (MSMR) 2007;14(5):2–7.

56. Department of Defense/Veterans Affairs. *Traumatic Brain Injury Planning Conference* [presentation]. National Conference Center, Lansdowne, VA, June 25–26, 2007.

94

57. Clark ME, Bair MJ, Buckenmaier CC 3rd, Gironda RJ, Walker RL. Pain and combat injuries in soldiers returning from Operations Enduring Freedom and Iraqi Freedom: Implications for research and practice. *J Rehabil Res Dev.* 2007;44(2):179–194.

58. Slomine BS, McCarthy ML, Ding R, et al. Health care utilization and needs after pediatric traumatic brain injury. *Pediatrics.* 2006;117(4):e663–e674.

59. Gironda RJ, Clark ME, Massengale JP, Walker RL. Pain among veterans of Operations Enduring Freedom and Iraqi Freedom. *Pain Med.* 2006;7(4):339–343.

60. Taber K, Warden D, Hurley R. Blast-related traumatic brain injury: What is known? *J Neuropsychiatr Clin Neurosci.* 2006;18:141–145.

61. Salter M, Woolf C. Cellular and molecular mechanisms of central sensitization. In: Hunt S. Koltzenburg M, eds. *The Neurobiology of Pain (Molecular and Cellular Biology).* Oxford, UK: Oxford University Press; 2005.

62. Carofoli E, Klee C. *Calcium as a Cellular Regulator.* New York: Oxford University Press; 1999.

63. Shipton EA, Tait B. Flagging the pain: Preventing the burden of chronic pain by identifying and treating risk factors in acute pain. *Eur J Anaesthesiol.* 2005;22(6):405–412.

64. Spiro A 3rd, Hankin CS, Mansell D, Kazis LE. Posttraumatic stress disorder and health status: The veterans health study. *J Ambul Care Manage.* 2006;29(1):71–86.

65. Giordano J. Understanding pain as disease and illness: Part one. *Pract. Pain Manage* 2006;6(6):70-73.

66. icasualties.org. Operation Iraqi Freedom. Online document at: www.icasualties.org/Iraq/Iraqideaths.aspx Accessed October 24, 2011.

67. Giordano J. Changing the practice of pain medicine writ large and small through identifying problems and establishing goals. *Pain Phys.* 2006;9(4):283–285.

68. Barnes PM, Bloom B, Nahin RL. Complementary and alternative medicine use among adults and children: United States, 2007. *Natl Health Stat Report.* 2008(12):1-23.

69. McPherson F, Schwenka MA. Use of complementary and alternative therapies among active duty soldiers, military retirees, and family members at a military hospital. *Mil Med.* 2004;169(5):354–357.

70. Klemm Analysis Group. *Alternative Medicine Therapy: Assessment of Current VHA Practices and Opportunities.* Washington, DC: Klemm Group; 1999.

71. Rick C, Feldman J. *Survey of Complementary and Alternative Medicine (CAM).* Washington, DC: Department of Veterans Affairs Health Administration, Office of Policy and planning. Healthcare Analysis and Information Group, 2002.

72. Kroesen K, Baldwin CM, Brooks AJ, Bell IR. US military veterans' perceptions of the conventional medical care system and their use of complementary and alternative medicine. *Fam Pract.* 2002;19(1):57–64.

73. Levine EG, Eckhardt J, Targ E. Change in post-traumatic stress symptoms following psychosocial treatment for breast cancer. *Psycho-oncology.* 2005;14(8):618–635.

74. Ai AL, Park CL. Possibilities of the positive following violence and trauma: Informing the coming decade of research. *J Interpers Violence.* 2005;20(2):242–250.

75. Osuch E, Engel CC Jr. Research on the treatment of trauma spectrum responses: The role of the optimal healing environment and neurobiology. *J Altern Complement Med.* 2004;10(suppl1):S211–S221.

76. Gordon JS, Staples JK, Blyta A, Bytyqi M. Treatment of posttraumatic stress disorder in postwar Kosovo high school students using mind–body skills groups: A pilot study. *J Trauma Stress.* 2004;17(2):143–147.

77. Benson H, Greenwood MM, Klemchuk H. The relaxation response: Psychophysiologic aspects and clinical applications. *Int J Psychiatry Med.* 1975;6(1–2):87–98.

78. Grossman P, Niemann L, Schmidt S, Walach H. Mindfulness-based stress reduction and health benefits: A meta-analysis. *J Psychosom Res.* 2004;57(1):35–43.

79. Raub JA. Psychophysiologic effects of Hatha Yoga on musculoskeletal and cardiopulmonary function: A literature review. *J Altern Complement Med.* 2002;8(6):797–812.

80. Niemtzow RC. Battlefield Acupuncture. *Med Acupunct.* 2007;19(4)225–228.

81. Goertz C, Niemtzow R, Burns S, Fritts M, Crawford C, Jonas WB. Auricular acupuncture in the treatment of acute pain syndromes: A pilot study. *Mil Med.* 2006;171(10):1010–1014.

82. Cutler MJ, Holland BS, Stupski BA, Gamber RG, Smith ML. Cranial manipulation can alter sleep latency and sympathetic nerve activity in humans: A pilot study. *J Altern Complement Med.* 2005;11(1):103–108.

83. Beal MW. Acupuncture and Oriental body work: Traditional and biomedical concepts in holistic care. History and basic concepts. *Holist Nurs Pract.* 2000;14(3):69–78.

84. Helms J. *Acupuncture Energetics: A Clinical Approach for Physicians.* Berkeley: Medical Acupuncture Publishers; 1996.

85. Eisenberg DM, Davis RB, Ettner SL, et al. Trends in alternative medicine use in the United States, 1990–1997: Results of a follow-up national survey. *JAMA.* 1998;280(18):1569–1575.

86. Green S, Buchbinder R, Hetrick S. Acupuncture for shoulder pain. *Cochrane Database Syst Rev.* 2005;2:CD005319.

87. Kalavapalli R, Singareddy R. Role of acupuncture in the treatment of insomnia: A comprehensive review. *Complement Ther Clin Pract.* 2007;13(3):184–193.

88. Lim B, Manheimer E, Lao L, Ziea E, Wisniewski J, Liu J, Berman B. Acupuncture for treatment of irritable bowel syndrome. *Cochrane Database Syst Rev.* 2006;4:CD005111.

89. Pilkington K, Kirkwood G, Rampes H, Cummings M, Richardson J. Acupuncture for anxiety and anxiety disorders—a systematic literature review. *Acupunct Med.* 2007;25 (1–2):1–10.

90. Smith CA, Hay PP. Acupuncture for depression. *Cochrane Database Syst Rev.* 2005;2:CD004046.

91. White A, Foster NE, Cummings M, Barlas P. Acupuncture treatment for chronic knee pain: A systematic review. *Rheumatology (Oxford).* 2007;46(3):384–390.

92. Martin DP, Sletten CD, Williams BA, Berger IH. Improvement in fibromyalgia symptoms with acupuncture: Results of a randomized controlled trial. *Mayo Clin Proc.* 2006;81(6):749–757.

93. Qu F, Zhou J. Electro-acupuncture in relieving labor pain. *Evid Based Complement Alternat Med.* 2007;4(1):125–130.

94. Usichenko TI, Hermsen M, Witstruck T, Hofer A, Pavlovic D, Lehmann C, Feyerherd F. Auricular acupuncture for pain relief after ambulatory knee arthroscopy—a pilot study. *Evid Based Complement Alternat Med.* 2005;2(2):185-189.

95. Pomeranz B. Acupuncture analgesia: Basic research. In: Stux G, Hammerschlag R, eds. *Clinical Acupuncture: Scientific Basis.* Berlin: Springer; 2001:1-28.

96. Lee A, Done ML. Stimulation of the wrist acupuncture point P6 for preventing postoperative nausea and vomiting. *Cochrane Database Syst Rev.* 2004;3:CD003281.

97. Allen J, Schnyer R, Hitt S. The efficacy of acupuncture in the treatment of major depression in women. *Psychol Sci.* 1998;9(5):397-401.

98. Blitzer L, Atchinson-Nevel D, Kenny M. Using acupuncture to treat major depressive disorder: A pilot investigation. *Clin Acupunct Oriental Med.* 2004;4(4):144-147.

99. Eich H, Agelink MW, Lehmann E, Lemmer W, Klieser E. Acupuncture in patients with minor depressive episodes and generalized anxiety: Results of an experimental study [in German]. *Fortsch Neurol Psychiatr.* 2000;68(3):137-144.

100. Han C, Li X, Lou H, Zhao X, Li X. Clinical study on electroacupuncture treatment for 30 cases of mental depression. *J Tradit Chin Med.* 2004;24:172-176.

101. Kober A, Scheck T, Schubert B, et al. Auricular acupressure as a treatment for anxiety in prehospital transport settings. *Anesthesiology.* 2003;98(6):1328-1332.

102. Manber R, Schnyer RN, Allen JJ, Rush AJ, Blasey CM. Acupuncture: A promising treatment for depression during pregnancy. *J Affect Disord.* 2004;83(1):89-95.

103. Ng M. The effectiveness of Traditional Chinese Medicine on depressive symptoms. *Diss Abstr Int B Sci Eng.* 1999;60:0860.

104. Roschke J, Wolf C, Muller MJ, et al. The benefit from whole body acupuncture in major depression. *J Affect Disord.* 2000;57(1-3):73-81.

105. Schnyer RN, Allen J. *Acupuncture in the Treatment of Depression: A Manual for Practice and Research.* London: Churchill-Livingstone; 2001.

106. Yang X, Liu X, Lou H, Jia Y. Clinical observation on needling extrachannel points in treating mental depression. *J Tradit Chin Med.* 1994;14(1):14-18.

107. Chan J, Briscomb D, Waterhouse E, Cannaby AM. An uncontrolled pilot study of HT7 for "stress." *Acupunct Med.* 2002;20(2-3):74-77.

108. Fassoulaki A, Paraskeva A, Patris K, Pourgiezi T, Kostopanagiotou G. Pressure applied on the Extra 1 acupuncture point reduces bispectral index values and stress in volunteers. *Anesth Analg.* 2003;96(3):885-890.

109. Wang JD, Kuo TB, Yang CC. An alternative method to enhance vagal activities and suppress sympathetic activities in humans. *Auton Neurosci.* 2002;100(1-2):90-95.

110. Chen A. An introduction to sequential electric acupuncture (SEA) in the treatment of stress related physical and mental disorders. *Acupunct Electrother Res.* 1992;17(4):273-283.

111. Middlekauff HR, Hui K, Yu JL, et al. Acupuncture inhibits sympathetic activation during mental stress in advanced heart failure patients. *J Card Fail.* 2002;8(6):399-406.

112. Montakab H. Acupuncture and insomnia [in German]. *Forsch Komplementarmed.* 1999;6(suppl 1):29-31.

113. Phillips KD, Skelton WD. Effects of individualized acupuncture on sleep quality in HIV disease. *J Assoc Nurses AIDS Care.* 2001;12(1):27-39.

114. Sok SR, Erlen JA, Kim KB. Effects of acupuncture therapy on insomnia. *J Adv Nurs.* 2003;44(4):375-384.

115. Spence DW, Kayumov L, Chen A, et al. Acupuncture increases nocturnal melatonin secretion and reduces insomnia and anxiety: A preliminary report. *J Neuropsychiatry Clin Neurosci.* 2004;16(1):19-28.

116. Audette JF, Ryan AH. The role of acupuncture in pain management. *Phys Med Rehabil Clin North Am.* 2004;15(4):v,749-772.

117. Birch S, Hesselink JK, Jonkman FA, Hekker TA, Bos A. Clinical research on acupuncture: Part 1. What have reviews of the efficacy and safety of acupuncture told us so far? *J Altern Complement Med.* 2004;10(1):468-480.

118. Ezzo J, Berman B, Hadhazy VA, Jadad AR, Lao L, Singh BB. Is acupuncture effective for the treatment of chronic pain? A systematic review. *Pain.* 2000;86(3):217-225.

119. Guerra de Hoyos JA, Andrés Martín M del C, Bassas y Baena de Leon E, Vigára Lopez M, Molina López T, Verdugo Morilla FA, González Moreno MJ. Randomised trial of long term effect of acupuncture for shoulder pain. *Pain.* 2004;112(3):289-298.

120. Melchart D, Linde K, Fischer P, White A, Allais G, Vickers A, Berman B. Acupuncture for recurrent headaches: A systematic review of randomized controlled trials. *Cephalalgia.* 1999;19(9):779-786;discussion:765.

121. Molsberger AF, Mau J, Pawelec DB, Winkler J. Does acupuncture improve the orthopedic management of chronic low back pain—a randomized, blinded, controlled trial with 3 months follow up. *Pain.* Oct 2002;99(3):579-587.

122. National Acupuncture Detoxification Association. Online document at: www.acudetox.com Accessed November 20, 2011.

123. Wu HM, Tang JL, Lin XP, Lau J, Leung PC, Woo J, Li YP. Acupuncture for stroke rehabilitation. *Cochrane Database Syst Rev.* 2006;3:CD004131.

124. Hollifield M, Sinclair-Lian N, Warner TD, Hammerschlag R. Acupuncture for posttraumatic stress disorder: A randomized controlled pilot trial. *J Nerv Ment Dis.* 2007;195(6):504-513.

125. Manheimer E, Linde K, Lao L, Bouter LM, Berman BM. Meta-analysis: Acupuncture for osteoarthritis of the knee. *Ann Intern Med.* 2007;146(12):868-877.

126. Cummings M. Myofascial pain from pectoralis major following trans-axillary surgery. *Acupunct Med.* 2003;21(3):105-107.

127. Donnellan CP. Acupuncture for central pain affecting the ribcage following traumatic brain injury and rib fractures—a case report. *Acupunct Med.* 2006;24(3):129-133.

128. Kober A, Scheck T, Greher M, et al. Prehospital analgesia with acupressure in victims of minor trauma: A prospective, randomized, double-blinded trial. *Anesth Analg.* 2002;95(3):723-727.

129. Li Y, Wang X, Li T. Acupuncture therapy for 12 cases of cranial trauma. *J Tradit Chin Med.* 1993;13(1):5-9.

130. Niemtzow RC, Gambel J, Helms J, Pock A, Burns SM, Baxter J. Integrating ear and scalp acupuncture techniques into the care of blast-injured United States military service

97

members with limb loss. *J Altern Complement Med.* 2006; 12(7):596-599.

131. Tkachuk VN, Medvedev IP, Bachurin EP. Effectiveness of acupuncture analgesia in the treatment of chronic post-traumatic pain syndromes [in Russian]. *Ortop Travmatol Protez.* 1991(5):33-35.

132. Haake M, Müller HH, Schade-Brittinger C, et al. German Acupuncture Trials (GERAC) for chronic low back pain: Randomized, multicenter, blinded, parallel-group trial with 3 groups. *Arch Intern Med.* 2007;167(17):1892-1898.

133. Witt C, Brinkhaus B, Jena S, et al. Acupuncture in patients with osteoarthritis of the knee: A randomised trial. *Lancet.* 2005;366(9480):136-143.

134. Hull SK, Page CP, Skinner BD, Linville JC, Coeytaux RR. Exploring outcomes associated with acupuncture. *J Altern Complement Med.* 2006;12(3):247 254.

135. Linde K, Streng A, Jurgens S, et al. Acupuncture for patients with migraine: A randomized controlled trial. *JAMA.* 2005;293(17):2118-2125.

136. Napadow V, Makris N, Liu J, Kettner NW, Kwong KK, Hui KK. Effects of electroacupuncture versus manual acupuncture on the human brain as measured by fMRI. *Hum Brain Mapp.* 2005;24(3):193-205.

137. Shen J. Research on the neurophysiological mechanisms of acupuncture: Review of selected studies and methodological issues. *J Altern Complement Med.* 2001;7(suppl1):S121-S127.

138. Ulett GA, Han S, Han JS. Electroacupuncture: Mechanisms and clinical application. *Biol Psychiatr.* 1998;44(2):129-138.

139. Cho Z-H, Son Y-D, Han J-H, Wong EK, et al. fMRI neurophysiological evidence of acupuncture mechanisms. *Med Acupunct.* 2002;14(1):16-22.

140. Li P, Pitsillides KF, Rendig SV, Pan HL, Longhurst JC. Reversal of reflex-induced myocardial ischemia by median nerve stimulation a feline model of electroacupuncture. *Circulation.* 1998;97(12):1186-1194.

141. Guo ZL, Moazzami AR, Longhurst JC. Stimulation of cardiac sympathetic afferents activates glutamatergic neurons in the parabrachial nucleus: Relation to neurons containing nNOS. *Brain Res.* 2005;1053(1-2):97-107.

142. Hui KK, Liu J, Makris N, et al. Acupuncture modulates the limbic system and subcortical gray structures of the human brain: Evidence from fMRI studies in normal subjects. *Hum Brain Mapp.* 2000;9(1):13-25.

143. Kong J, Ma L, Gollub RL, et al. A pilot study of functional magnetic resonance imaging of the brain during manual and electroacupuncture stimulation of acupuncture point (LI-4 Hegu) in normal subjects reveals differential brain activation between methods. *J Altern Complement Med.* Aug 2002;8(4):411-419.

144. Birch S. A review and analysis of placebo treatments, placebo effects, and placebo controls in trials of medical procedures when sham is not inert. *J Altern Complement Med.* 2006;12(3):303-310.

145. Hammerschlag R. Methodological and ethical issues in clinical trials of acupuncture. *J Altern Complement Med.* 1998;4(2):159-171.

146. Itaya K, Manaka Y, Ohkubo C, Asano M. Effects of acupuncture needle application upon cutaneous microcircula-

tion of rabbit ear lobe. *Acupunct Electrother Res.* 1987; 12(1):45-51.

147. Litscher G. Bioengineering assessment of acupuncture, part 2: Monitoring of microcirculation. *Crit Rev Biomed Eng.* 2006;34(4):273-294.

148. Bing Z, Cesselin F, Bourgoin S, Clot AM, Hamon M, Le Bars D. Acupuncture-like stimulation induces a heterosegmental release of Met-enkephalin-like material in the rat spinal cord. *Pain.* 1991;47(1):71-77.

149. Murase K, Kawakita K. Diffuse noxious inhibitory controls in anti-nociception produced by acupuncture and moxibustion on trigeminal caudalis neurons in rats. *Jpn J Physiol.* Feb 2000;50(1):133-140.

150. Avants SK, Margolin A, Holford TR, Kosten TR. A randomized controlled trial of auricular acupuncture for cocaine dependence. *Arch Intern Med.* 2000;160(15):2305-2312.

151. Margolin A, Avants SK, Kleber HD. Rationale and design of the Cocaine Alternative Treatments Study (CATS): A randomized, controlled trial of acupuncture. *J Altern Complement Med.* 1998;4(4):405-418.

152. Langevin HM, Churchill DL, Fox JR, Badger GJ, Garra BS, Krag MH. Biomechanical response to acupuncture needling in humans. *J Appl Physiol.* 2001;91(6):2471-2478.

153. Brinkhaus B, Witt CM, Jena S, et al. Acupuncture in patients with chronic low back pain: A randomized controlled trial. *Arch Intern Med.* 2006;166(4):450-457.

154. Diener HC, Kronfeld K, Boewing G, et al. Efficacy of acupuncture for the prophylaxis of migraine: A multicentre randomised controlled clinical trial. *Lancet Neurol.* 2006; 5(4):310-316.

155. Kleinhenz J, Streitberger K, Windeler J, Gussbacher A, Mavridis G, Martin E. Randomised clinical trial comparing the effects of acupuncture and a newly designed placebo needle in rotator cuff tendinitis. *Pain.* Nov 1999;83(2):235-241.

156. Park J, White A, Stevinson C, Ernst E, James M. Validating a new non-penetrating sham acupuncture device: Two randomised controlled trials. *Acupunct Med.* 2002;20(4):168-174.

157. Langevin HM, Hammerschlag R, Lao L, Napadow V, Schnyer RN, Sherman KJ. Controversies in acupuncture research: Selection of controls and outcome measures in acupuncture clinical trials. *J Altern Complement Med.* 2006; 12(10):943 953.

158. Hammerschlag R, Zwickey H. Evidence-based complementary and alternative medicine: Back to basics. *J Altern Complement Med.* 2006;12(4):349-350.

159. Moerman D, Jonas W. Deconstructing the placebo effect and finding the meaning response. *Ann Intern Med.* 2002;136:471 476.

Address correspondence to:
Wayne B. Jonas, MD
Samueli Institute,
1737 King Street, Suite 600
Alexandria VA 22314

E-mail: wjonas@siib.org

Chairman SANDERS. Thank you very much, Dr. Kahn.
Dr. Edlund.

STATEMENT OF MARK EDLUND, M.D., Ph.D., SENIOR RESEARCH PUBLIC HEALTH ANALYST, BEHAVIORAL HEALTH EPIDEMIOLOGY PROGRAM, RTI INTERNATIONAL

Dr. EDLUND. Good morning. Thank you for inviting me. My name is Mark Edlund, and I am a health services researcher at RTI International and a practicing psychiatrist.

For the past 10 years my colleagues and I have researched patterns of opioid painkiller prescribing in Blue Cross/Blue Shield, Arkansas Medicaid, and more recently the VA.

Our research involves analyzing administrative data and pharmacy records. Most recently, our research has focused on national patterns of opioid prescribing in the VA, supported by a grant from the National Institute of Drug Abuse.

The VA data come from the years 2009 to 2011. My testimony today will provide initial findings from our NIDA-funded work. This work examined three aspects of opioid prescribing in the VA.

One, rates of opioid prescribing in VA patients with chronic non-cancer pain. Two, factors associated with discontinuation of chronic opioid therapy. And, three, factors associated with heavy utilization of opioids among VA patients with chronic pain.

Rates of opioid prescribing in VA patients with chronic pain. Many VA patients have chronic pain, most commonly back pain and arthritis. Our results suggest that, among VA patients with chronic non-cancer pain who are using VA services at least twice per year, a little over half receive at least one outpatient opioid prescription in that year.

Although comparing rates of opioid use between health care systems can be imprecise, this rate is approximately the same rate as found in other health care systems and in other health care plans.

VA patients with chronic pain who receive opioids have a median of about 120 days of use in a year, that is, they used opioids about one 1 of 3 days—the median individual. This is generally higher than in other health care systems.

In this same VA cohort, the median daily opioid dose is modest, about 21 milligram morphine equivalents. So, morphine equivalents are the way we standardize all these different opioids, and 21 milligrams is fairly low. High would be thought of as, say, 120 to 200. So, the median dose is generally lower in the VA than in other health care systems.

Of the VA chronic pain patients prescribed opioids, the percentage who receive high doses of opioids is relatively small, about 5 percent. This is also lower than in other health care systems. This is important because high dose is an important predictor of adverse outcomes.

The opioid use of OEF/OIF VA patients has been the subject of scrutiny. We found that, among VA patients with chronic pain, OEF/OIF patients were less likely to be prescribed opioids as compared to other VA patients; and among VA patients with chronic pain who were prescribed opioids, OEF/OIF veterans were less likely to be heavy utilizers of opioids.

Rates of opioid discontinuation. Among VA patients who received at least 90 days of VA opioids within a 180-day period in 2009, we looked at rates of discontinuation where discontinuation was defined as 6 months with no opioid prescription.

We found that among these VA patients nearly 80 percent will receive years of opioid therapy. This is consistent with what we have found in analyses of other health care plans. While high daily doses is not common among VA patients, both high daily doses and use of long-acting opioids were strong predictors of opioid discontinuation, or excuse me, continuation.

Individuals with substance abuse disorders and mental health disorders were more likely to discontinue opioids in the VA. This is important because these patients are those who are at increased risk for opioid abuse.

Factors associated with heavy opioid utilization among VA patients. In analyses of data from other health systems show individuals with substance abuse disorders are at a high risk for heavy utilization of opioids.

However, in an analysis of VA patients with chronic pain known to be using the VA at least twice in a fiscal year, individuals with substance abuse were less likely to be heavy utilizers of opiates.

In summary, while comparing health care systems can be imprecise, we found, one, among chronic pain patients rates of any opioid use is approximately the same in the VA and non-VA systems.

However, among chronic pain patients in VA who receive opiates, the number of days for which they received opioids in a given year is generally higher than in non-VA systems. However, median daily dose in the VA is lower than in other health care systems.

Finally, it appears that the VA does a better job of screening out individuals with substance abuse and mental health disorders from heavy utilization of opioids which is also very important because those are the people who are most likely to go on to abuse.

[The prepared statement of Dr. Edlund follows:]

PREPARED STATEMENT OF MARK J. EDLUND, M.D., PH.D., SENIOR RESEARCH PUBLIC HEALTH ANALYST, BEHAVIORAL HEALTH EPIDEMIOLOGY PROGRAM, RTI INTERNATIONAL

Good morning, thank you for inviting me. My name is Mark Edlund. I am a health services researcher at RTI International, and a practicing psychiatrist. For the past 10 years my colleagues and I have researched patterns of opioid painkiller prescribing in different health care systems. Our research involves analyzing administrative data and pharmacy records. Most recently, our research has focused on national patterns of opioid prescribing in the VHA, supported by a grant from the National Institute of Drug Abuse (NIDA).

My testimony today will provide initial findings from our NIDA-funded work. This work examined three aspects of opioid prescribing in the VHA: rates of opioid prescribing in VHA patients with chronic noncancer pain; factors associated with discontinuation of chronic opioid therapy; and, factors associated with chronic opioid use among VHA patients.

Our research used VHA administrative and pharmacy data from years 2009 to 2011. We have thus far conducted three different analyses of this data. The results from those analyses were reported at the Addiction Health Services meetings held October, 2013 in Portland, Oregon and the American Academy of Pain Medicine meetings held March, 2014 in Phoenix, Arizona.

While some of the research methods were the same for all three studies, some methods varied in each study, as did the VHA patient sample.

METHODS FOR ALL ANALYSES

Data Source

We used data from three VHA Sources
• Pharmacy Benefits Management Service (PBM)
• VHA Corporate Data Warehouse
• OEF/OIF roster

Opioid Use Variables. Data included all opioid prescriptions (including date, daily dose, and type of opioid), other than injectable opioids and opioid suppositories (due to lack of conversion factors). We recorded the total number of opioid prescription fills for each patient within the fiscal year and calculated the number of days supplied for each patient in the year, as recorded by the dispensing pharmacist. The mean dose in morphine equivalents per day supplied for each patient was calculated by summing the morphine equivalents for each prescription filled during the year, and dividing by the number of days supplied.

Other Variables. We used International Classification of Diseases–9th Revision (ICD–9) codes from VHA Corporate Data Warehouse to construct variables for mental health diagnoses and substance use disorders. Chronic non-cancer pain conditions were also identified through ICD–9 codes and grouped into five broad categories encompassing the most common chronic noncancer pain conditions. These groupings included neck pain, back pain, arthritis/joint pain, headache/migraine and neuropathic pain, which are common to VHA patients. Demographic information such as age, race, gender and marital status were also extracted from the VHA Corporate Data Warehouse.

IRB Approval. All analyses were approved by the Institutional Review Boards of The Central Arkansas Veterans Healthcare System and the University of Arkansas for Medical Sciences. A data use agreement was executed with each data repository.

ANALYSIS 1—PATTERNS OF OPIOID USE FOR CHRONIC NONCANCER PAIN

Study Sample

The study sample consisted of VHA patients in years 2009 to 2011 who met the following criteria. INCLUSION CRITERIA: 1) chronic noncancer pain diagnosis, as defined by two clinical encounters for the same chronic noncancer pain condition (neck pain, back pain, arthritis, headache/migraine, or neuropathic pain) at least 30 days apart, but no more than 365 days apart, 2) Received at least one opioid prescription during the year of chronic noncancer pain diagnosis, 3) Age 18 or older. EXCLUSION CRITERIA: 1) Cancer diagnosis at any time in 2008–12 other than non-melanoma skin cancer, 2) resident of VHA nursing home or living in VHA domiciliary, 3) enrolled in VHA hospice benefits, 4) incomplete opioid prescription data, or 5) a prescription for a parenteral, suppository, or trans mucosal opioid. These criteria allow us to focus on VHA patients likely receiving opioids for the treatment of chronic noncancer pain.

KEY RESULTS FROM FIRST ANALYSES

Many VHA patients have chronic pain, with the most common sources being back pain and arthritis. Our results suggest that, among VHA patients with chronic noncancer pain who are using the VA at least twice per year, a little over half receive at least one outpatient opioid prescription in that year. VA patients with chronic pain who receive opioids have a median of 120 days of use in a year, or about one out of three days. In this same VHA cohort the median daily opioid dose is modest, about 21 milligram morphine equivalents. 21 milligram morphine equivalents is fairly low, equivalent to about 2 Vicodin tablets. In our analyses the percentage of VHA patients who received high doses of opioids was relatively small—about five percent. Among VHA patients with chronic noncancer pain, 44% of all opioids were used by just 5% of patients; 1% of patients accounted for 17% of all opioids utilized.

The opioid use of OEF/OIF VHA patients has been the subject of scrutiny. We found that, among VHA patients with chronic noncancer pain, OEF/OIF patients were less likely to be prescribed opioids compared to non OEF/OIF VHA patients, and less likely to be heavy utilizers of opioids.

Conclusions: About half of all VHA patients with chronic noncancer pain receive opioids, and among those who receive opioids, the median days of use is 120 days. The median daily dose is modest. Total opioid use is heavily concentrated among a relatively small proportion of the VHA population with chronic noncancer pain.

Second Analysis:

Our second set of analyses focused on discontinuation from chronic opioid therapy.

ANALYSIS 2—DISCONTINUATION FROM CHRONIC OPIOID THERAPY

Study Sample

The study sample consisted of all adult VHA patients receiving 90 days or greater supply of non-parenteral opioids with less than a 30-day gap in supply within a 180-day period between January 1, 2009 and December 31, 2011. We refer to individuals who met these inclusion criteria as receiving chronic opioid therapy. The index date was defined as the first day of this 90-day period. A minimum of two prior encounters in the year preceding the index date were required to document routine use of VHA care. The year preceding the index period was used to identify additional exclusionary criteria and relevant co-variables. Veterans with an ICD–9 cancer diagnosis (with the exception of non-melanoma skin cancers) and administrative codes for VHA nursing home use, hospice or palliative care services in the 360 days before and after the index date were excluded. Additionally, veterans with incomplete opioid prescription data (unknown dosages or types) or enrollment in a methadone maintenance program or receiving buprenorphine at any time were excluded.

Given high rates of interrupted or episodic use among chronic opioid users and to maintain consistency in definitions, discontinuation was defined as the first run-out day of a minimum 180-day period with no opioid prescriptions. In order to distinguish clearly between disenrollment from VHA and opioid discontinuation, participants without any VHA services use in the 90 days after discontinuation were excluded.

If any two prescriptions overlapped by greater than 20% or greater than ten days, the overlapping portions of the prescription were assumed to be taken concurrently and the overlapping days were only included once in the opioid days calculation. If the overlap was ≤20% and ≤10 days the second prescription was shifted and the overlapping days from both the first and second prescription were included in the opioid days calculation. A dichotomous variable for the presence of multiple opioids defined as two or more types of opioids that overlapped by more than 30 days in any 40-day period was created as a surrogate for potential opioid misuse.

VHA service utilization during the period of chronic opioid therapy was calculated as the total number of mental health encounters, substance use encounters and all other VHA encounters abstracted from Current Procedural Terminology (CPT) codes in the 90 days post-index.

KEY RESULTS FROM ANALYSIS 2—DISCONTINUATION FROM CHRONIC OPIOID THERAPY

We identified 814,311 VHA patients who met our criteria for chronic opioid therapy. After exclusions were applied, 550,548 (67.6% of chronic opioid users) were eligible for analysis and 542,843 were entered into the statistical models. (We excluded 7,705 (1.4%) of the sample due to missing data, primarily the absence of reliable rural/urban coding). The sample was primarily male (93%), white (74%) and urban-dwelling (68%), with a mean age of 57.8 years and 52% were married. At one year after their index prescription date, only 7.5% of the sample had discontinued chronic opioid therapy.

The majority of the sample suffered from at least one chronic noncancer pain condition (82.3%); just over a quarter of the sample had two chronic noncancer pain conditions (26.7%). Similarly, 62.3% of the sample had a mental health diagnosis, the most common being depressive disorder (29.7%). Only 14.5% of the sample had a substance use disorder, while 25.6% of the total sample used tobacco. The mean number of total clinical encounters in 90-days post-index was almost 9 (mean 8.92, SD 11.01).

The mean daily morphine equivalent dose was 40.7 mg (SD 61.67 mg) among the VHA patients in this analysis though the median was 26 mg and only 7% received greater than 100 mg daily morphine equivalent. Nearly all received short-acting opioids (97.1%). Only 12.3% received multiple concurrent opioid prescriptions, usually a long-acting plus a short-acting opioid, and over half (57%) had received greater than 90 days total opioid supply in the year preceding their index date.

We conducted analyses to examine factors associated with discontinuation from long-term opioid therapy. The maximum time available for follow-up was 1,279 days (3.5 years), and of those who discontinued (20%, N=110,460), the mean time to discontinuation was 530 days (SD 298.15, median: 465). The majority of the sample continued use through the end of the follow-up period. Demographic characteristics associated with higher rates of discontinuation of long-term opioid therapy included being younger or older than VHA patients aged 50–65 (0–30 years HR=1.52, 95% CI 1.47 to 1.57 and >65 years HR=1.34, 95% CI 1.32 to 1.36), non-married status (HR 1.06, 95% CI 1.05 to 1.08) and African American race (HR 1.04, 95% CI 1.02 to 1.06). Compared with VHA patients living in an isolated rural setting, those in an urban setting were significantly more likely to discontinue long-term opioid therapy (HR 1.08, 95% CI 1.05 to 1.10).

VHA patients who were receiving higher average daily doses of opioids were less likely to discontinue chronic opioid therapy. Those taking long-acting opioid formulations had roughly 6% lower rates discontinuation of chronic opioid therapy compared with those taking short-acting opioid medications. (HR 0.94, 95% CI 0.90 to 0.98 VHA patients). Those receiving multiple opioid prescriptions concurrently had about a 20% lower rate of discontinuation compared with VHA patients receiving only one opioid medication (HR 0.80, 95% CI 0.78 to 0.82). Finally, VHA patients with significant use of opioids in the year prior to the index date had almost a 30% lower rate of opioid discontinuations (HR 0.69, 95% CI 0.68 to 0.70). VHA patients who had multiple types of pain or who had greater level of medical comorbidity were more likely to continue chronic opioid therapy.

For the cohort of VHA patients in this analysis, mental health diagnoses were associated with greater likelihood of discontinuation of chronic opioid therapy, with schizophrenia and bipolar diagnoses associated with nearly 20% greater hazard of discontinuation (HR 1.20, 95% CI 1.16 to 1.25 for schizophrenia and HR 1.20, 95% CI 1.16 to 1.23 for bipolar). Alcohol use disorder (HR 1.10, 95% CI 1.07 to 1.12), opioid use disorder (HR 1.09, 95% CI 1.06 to 1.13) and non-opioid use disorders (HR 1.22, 95% CI 1.19 to 1.25) were all significantly associated with higher rates of discontinuation. In contrast to other mental health and substance use predictors, tobacco use disorders were associated with higher rates of continued long-term opioid therapy (HR 0.96, 95% CI 0.94 to 0.97).

Conclusions: Among VHA patients who had received at least 90 days of opioids within a 180 day period in 2009, nearly 80% went on to receive years of opioid therapy. This is similar in other health care plans. However, in other health care plans we studied, individuals who were at high risk for opioid abuse, namely those with substance use disorders and mental health disorders, were more likely to receive high dose opioids and less likely to discontinue opioids. We generally did not find this in the VHA. As noted above, VHA patients with mental health diagnoses, diagnosed disorders related to alcohol use as well as opioid and non-opioid substance use disorders were more likely to be discontinued from long-term opioid therapy. Thus, it appears that VHA does better than other health care systems previously studied in terms of discontinuing patients from chronic opioid therapy.

Third Analysis:

Our third analysis examined factors associated with chronic opioid use among VHA patients who regularly used VHA care in FY 2011.

ANALYSIS 3—CHRONIC OPIOID USE AMONG ALL VHA PATIENTS WITH OR WITHOUT
CHRONIC NON CANCER PAIN

Study Sample

To be included in the cohort for the third analysis we identified all Veterans who had at least one outpatient opioid prescription in FY 2011 using data from the VHA Pharmacy Benefits Management Service. Similar to our 2nd analysis we used secure mechanisms to link the data from the Pharmacy Benefits Management Service to that of the Corporate Data Warehouse to identify VHA patients who used VHA care at least twice in FY 2011. VHA patients with an ICD–9 cancer diagnosis (with the exception of non-melanoma skin cancers) and administrative codes for VHA nursing home use, hospice or palliative care services, had codes for methadone maintenance or were receiving buprenorphine were also excluded from the sample. In addition, VHA patients receiving outpatient opioid prescriptions for injectable opioids, opioid suppositories or trans mucosal opioid preparations were also excluded from the analysis. VHA patients were not required to have a chronic pain diagnosis to be included in this sample. Based on these inclusion and exclusion criteria, we identified a total of 1,127,955 VHA patients who were using opioid medications in FY 2011. Almost 52% (584,765) of VHA patients in this analysis were using opioids for 91 or more days during that fiscal year.

KEY RESULTS FROM ANALYSIS 3—CHRONIC OPIOID USE AMONG ALL VHA PATIENTS WITH
OR WITHOUT CHRONIC NONCANCER PAIN

In unadjusted results, chronic opioid users were slightly older than non-chronic users (59 years vs 57 years), were more likely to be white (72.9% vs 65.9%), and were less likely to be OEF/OIF/OND Veterans (5.9% vs 11.1%).

We used a logistic regression model to identify factors associated with chronic opioid use in this cohort in FY 2011 (adjusted results). In this cohort, opioid use was most common in VHA patients ages 56 to 65 years; patients in other age groups were less likely to have chronic opioid use. The difference was most noticeable in the youngest age group. VHA patients ages 18–25 were almost 62% less likely than VHA patients ages 56–65 years to receive chronic opioid therapy (OR=0.38, 95% CI=.36–.39). Non-white VHA patients were approximately 28% less likely than white VHA patients to receive opioid medications chronically (OR=.72, 95% CI=.71–.73). VHA patients in whom race was unknown were also less likely to receive chronic opioid medications although the difference was less pronounced with these patients being 8% less likely to receive chronic opioid therapy compared with white patients (OR=.92, 95% CI=.90–.93). In this cohort women patients were 22% less likely to receive chronic opioid therapy compared with male patients (OR=.78, 95% CI=.77–.79). VHA patients who were identified as OEF/OIF Veterans were 34% less likely to receiving chronic opioid therapy compared with non-OEF/OIF Veterans (OR=.66, 95% CI=.65–.67).

103

In this cohort having PTSD or a depressive disorder was associated with receiving chronic opioid therapy. VHA patients in this cohort with a PTSD diagnosis were 16% more likely to receiving chronic opioid therapy compared with VHA patients without PTSD (OR=1.16, 95% CI=1.15–1.18). VHA patients in this cohort with a diagnosis of a depressive disorder were 25% more likely to receive chronic opioid medications (OR=1.25, 95% CI=1.24–1.26).

In this model, likelihood of chronic opioid use was most strongly associated with opioid dose, use of long-acting opioid medications and receiving multiple opioid medications concurrently. VHA patients in this cohort who were receiving 100MG morphine equivalent dose or more each day were 68% more likely to receive opioids chronically (OR=1.68, 95% CI=1.60–1.76. VHA patients who were receiving long-acting opioid medications were almost four times as likely to receive opioids chronically compared to those receiving short-acting medications (OR=3.77, 95% CI=3.6–3.8) while those receiving multiple opioid medications concurrently were more than 30 times more likely to receive opioids chronically (OR=30.8, 95% CI=29.4–32.3).

Conclusions: Of VHA patients who use opioids, about half use them chronically (at least 89 days per year). VHA patients who were non-whites, OEF/OIF, or female were less likely to receive chronic opioid therapy. Individuals with mental health disorders were more likely to receive opioids chronically, but the magnitude of this effect was small. Higher opioid dose, use of multiple opioids concurrently and use of long-acting opioid medications were strongly associated with chronic opioid use.

CAVEATS

Our results should be interpreted with 4 factors in mind. First, we had access only to VHA records, and do not know about opioids VHA patients may be receiving outside the VHA system. Second, the definition of chronic pain is inherently subjective. In our first analysis we used a definition that is relatively strict. With less strict definitions, the percentage of VA chronic pain patients receiving opioids would likely be lower, as would the number of days of opioids used in a year. Third, the definition of high dose opioids is also subjective. We used a measure of high dose opioids that is on the low side. If we had used a measure that was higher, then our estimate of the percentage of VA patients with chronic pain who received high dose opioid therapy would have been lower. Fourth, although we reviewed records of all VHA patients in various years we included only specific patients in our analyses because we wanted to identify Veterans that were known to be using VHA care regularly.

Thank you.

Chairman SANDERS. Dr. Edlund, thank you very much for your testimony.

Let me start with Dr. Kahn and just ask you a pretty simple question. Let's say there is a veteran who is coming back from Iraq and Afghanistan dealing with pain issues, back pain or whatever it may be, he or she has difficulty sleeping, maybe the marriage is in trouble, they have difficulty holding on to a job.

You said the issue here is not to deal with pain but to deal with the person. In the real world, somebody walks into your door with the issues I have described, the easy path is to medicate. Historically, we have done a lot of that. You have got pain; here are some drugs.

You are proposing a different way. In English and maybe some concrete examples, what does that mean? What do you do with that individual who walked in your door?

Ms. KAHN. So, I hope I made it clear that I am not suggesting an either/or approach.

Chairman SANDERS. No. We understand absolutely.

Ms. KAHN. OK. And I want to state clearly that I am not a physician.

Chairman SANDERS. Right.

Ms. KAHN. OK. So, that said, yes. I assume a physician would address issues of pain directly but at the same time because people's experience of pain and their capacity to handle and to cope with pain and manage whatever level of pain they are experiencing, is influenced by these other things like their general state of anxiety or whether or not they are sleep deprived and, therefore, on edge in a different way, we want to come up under them in terms of those elements of life at the same time as addressing the pain directly. That is what I am suggesting.

Chairman SANDERS. Give me some examples, if you can, of the effectiveness of the approach you are utilizing. Does it work? Do you have some examples of people who have walked in the door who have been able to get effective treatment, see real improvements in their lives with minimal use of heavy drugs?

Ms. KAHN. I think I am actually not in a position to answer that yet because in my own practice of offering Mission Reconnect to people the first trial with that program was not done in a VA context or in a medical context, thus I did not have access to medical records to be able to assess changes in medication prescription or use.

We have been approached by psychologists at the Tampa VA, and they are in the process of preparing a proposal to look at exactly that, to apply Mission Reconnect with other care for people who are both high PTSD and high pain.

Chairman SANDERS. OK. Dr. Edlund, do you have some thoughts on that?

Dr. EDLUND. I think that these strategies are underutilized. I think that they hold promise. I think that they are particularly attractive in that they are noninvasive and they do not involve medication.

I think that ultimately they are going to be an important part of the puzzle and there is no one piece of the puzzle that is dominant. So, I agree that all of these elements need to be brought to the fore.

Chairman SANDERS. In your opinion, Dr. Edlund, has VA been aggressive in exploring these new approaches?

Dr. EDLUND. I would say that the VA has been more aggressive than the rest of the American health care system and that the level of aggressiveness has markedly increased in the last 2 or 3 years.

Chairman SANDERS. So, if you walked into a VA facility you would be more likely to have the option of looking at these approaches than in a private-sector hospital. Is that what you are saying?

Dr. EDLUND. Yes, almost certainly.

Chairman SANDERS. OK. Dr. Kahn, do you have anything to add to that?

Ms. KAHN. Well, only that because in the non-governmental world, in the world of private insurance, most complementary and alternative medicine forms have not been and continue not to really be fully reimbursed. Then the patient is faced with a tougher choice if they are going to have to pay for it themselves in a private hospital than in the VA. So, I would imagine there would be greater use in the VA.

Chairman SANDERS. Well, that is an interesting observation. So, because insurance companies do not cover many of these complementary or alternative approaches, the private hospital is constrained about what kind of therapies it can offer.

Ms. KAHN. Not necessarily what ones they offer but how they offer them. An increasing percentage of private hospitals do offer them, sometimes paid for philanthropically. Sometimes the hospital itself will pay and often it will be a fee that the patients themselves have to absorb.

Chairman SANDERS. OK. Thank you very much.

Senator Burr.

Senator BURR. Mr. Chairman, thank you.

The one thing that I hope I will not fall prey to is trying to practice medicine from this side of the dias.

Chairman SANDERS. Give it a try.

[Laughter.]

Senator BURR. The truth is that the VA is a medical home and not everybody that prescribes in the private sector is necessarily that patient's medical home. They are referred to that pain specialist by their medical home and I think a medical home is more apt to look at all the conditions that surround an individual before they make a determination as to which course to follow, and I think that is why maybe in the private sector there are options.

I think the Chairman's intent was to say that they are not all paid for by their insurance company where we have expanded it greatly in the VA.

Dr. Kahn, I am fascinated to look at the studies once you have completed them in these multi-geographical areas with a variation of our active duty forces to see if we find variations between the Army and others. I look forward to that.

But you testified that the VA needs to change from a problem-fixing mentality to a more rounded approach toward health care, and I think you alluded to the fact that this is a big organization. There are a lot of people, and that makes it challenging.

What do you see as those challenges?

Ms. KAHN. Well, first of all, any big boat takes a while to turn. So, size is simply one problem. I do not know exactly what the level of acceptance right now is among providers across the VA so that would have to be assessed.

In general, I would say in the field of health care across all health care professions—complementary, alternative, conventional, I would say many of us are fairly arrogant about our own approach and not necessarily even well informed about other approaches.

Senator BURR. What do you see as the biggest impediment for VA making this transition?

Ms. KAHN. I do not see anything insurmountable. I think if the will is there it can absolutely be done. I think in general we have not seen large-scale use of integrative health care. It has been sort of an almost boutique form, but I think the single largest civilian health system that is integrating across the whole system is Allina Health, which is in Minnesota and Wisconsin. It is not the 150 medical centers and 1,500 clinics that the VA has. It is 12 hospitals and 150 clinics. But it begins to show the scalability, and I think the VA could do it.

Senator BURR. Dr. Edlund, tremendous research comes out of RTI, and we are grateful for that, and thank you for your work on this. Your testimony discusses several research studies you conducted regarding the patterns of opiate prescribing in VA facilities.

Let me ask you, does RTI plan to conduct further research in that area?

Dr. EDLUND. I am hoping to submit another grant, yes; and we have submitted grants in the past that have not been funded. So, yes, it is an active area of research.

Senator BURR. Can you describe for us what you see that next research project structured like, that you would submit that grant for?

Dr. EDLUND. Yes. The most recent grant that I have is actually not a VA grant. It is outside of the VA. Well, we will also be using VA physicians.

We are looking at what goes into or how do physicians arrive at the decision to prescribe an opiate. Opiates are a two-edged sword, and the question is always how do you balance the risks and benefits.

I am interested in understanding how they do that and what makes them decide along with the patient, OK, we are going to prescribe an opiate in this case or we are not going to prescribe an opiate in this case or we are going to escalate the opiate.

So, these kind of fundamental decision-making processes that the physicians have to make along with the patient, we really do not understand at all and our next grant is to go in and try to better understand that.

Senator BURR. Well, maybe, I can persuade Dr. Briggs for the Committee to answer that question that I believe she has probably looked at and it is a fascinating thing because I think we are making a big assumption that there is a tremendous amount of thought put into that determination.

My observation would be opiates are prescribed a lot of times because that is what the patient came in and asked for, and doctors feel compelled to send them out with what, in fact, they requested. That may be part of our problem.

I thank the Chair.

Chairman SANDERS. Thank you, Senator Burr.

Senator Blumenthal.

Senator BLUMENTHAL. Thank you, Mr. Chairman.

Dr. Edlund, this number may have been in your testimony but I have trouble seeing it highlighted there. Is there an average for the amount of time or the amount of drugs, opioids that are taken when they are prescribed?

Dr. EDLUND. I am sorry. I am not understanding. Is there what?

Senator BLUMENTHAL. Is there an average either period of time or amount of drugs over a period of time? In other words, someone who is prescribed an opioid takes it on average for 6 months, 2 weeks, a year.

Is there any data on how long the average prescription lasts?

Dr. EDLUND. Yes. Well, what we know is that—we differentiate between acute opiate use and chronic opiate use. So acute use would be you hurt your ankle and that is not what we are talking about.

But with chronic use, what we know is that once an individual has been on chronic opioids for about 90 days, then most of those individuals will go on to use opioids for years. Really, you know, we cannot figure out and an average because at the end of 5 years, 75 percent of them will still be on opiates.

Senator BLUMENTHAL. Is there any data on whether the prescription for chronic users increases over time? In other words, does the amount of opioids prescribed have to increase to, in effect, take care of the same level of pain or for some other reason?

Dr. EDLUND. No. That is a very good question and that is poorly understood, meaning whether or not in what percentage of cases the opioid dose can be stable.

Definitely in some cases you have to increase the dose over time because the patient develops a tolerance and that is the whole problem with opiate use is that, you know, it is a spiral that is always going upward. But we do not know how many people are in a spiral going upward and how many people are relatively stable.

Senator BLUMENTHAL. Is that not an important question?

Dr. EDLUND. Yes. There are a lot of fundamental important questions in opioids that have not been answered.

Senator BLUMENTHAL. I apologize for interrupting you but my time is limited; to follow up on Senator Burr's excellent question, it may well be that the patient comes in and says I need more, Doc.

Dr. EDLUND. It may very well be and I agree that a lot of times probably not a lot of thought is put into these decisions.

Senator BLUMENTHAL. And is there a way, for example, to have trip wires, for a lack of a better word? In other words, after 6 months there has to be a complete review by some independent medical professional or panel or some kind of authority to say, you know, there is a pattern here, increasing use over 6 months or, in other words, some kind of independent review.

Dr. EDLUND. Yes. Obviously that could be done easily, but to my knowledge it is fairly rarely done.

Senator BLUMENTHAL. And in your experience, to talk about Post Traumatic Stress—and I would ask this question of Dr. Kahn as well—Post Traumatic Stress, is that condition addressed therapeutically by opioid use or does opioid use address other conditions that, as Secretary Petzel said, may be found accompanied with Post Traumatic Stress, pain along with Post Traumatic Stress; is there an affect on the Post Traumatic Stress of using opioids either good or bad?

Dr. EDLUND. I am not familiar with that research. I do know that a lot of people with PTSD receive opioids, but I cannot speak to the finding.

Senator BLUMENTHAL. There is no research so far as you are aware——

Dr. EDLUND. Not that I am aware of.

Senator BLUMENTHAL [continuing]. Showing the effects on Post Traumatic Stress, minus of opioid use?

Dr. EDLUND. No, not that I am familiar with.

Senator BLUMENTHAL. Dr. Kahn, are you aware of any such research?

Ms. KAHN. No, I am not.

Senator BLUMENTHAL. I would welcome—since I cannot ask the past panel whether they are aware of such research, if they are, please make me and perhaps the Committee aware of it.

I thank you, Mr. Chairman. Just one footnote here which I have said before. I refer to Post Traumatic Stress as Post Traumatic Stress rather than Post Traumatic Stress Disorder, and I had said it to others who have testified here including Secretary Shinseki.

You may agree or disagree but I think it is important to remove the stigma of Post Traumatic Stress by not referring to it as a disorder. I may be clinically and medically out in left field but so be it. Thank you.

Thank you Mr. Chairman.

Chairman SANDERS. Senator Blumenthal, thank you very much and, Dr. Kahn, Dr. Edlund, thank you very much for helping us out on this very important issue.

Ms. KAHN. Thank you.

Chairman SANDERS. And with that, the hearing is now adjourned.

[Whereupon, at 11:53 a.m., the Committee was adjourned.]

APPENDIX

PREPARED STATEMENT OF THE AMERICAN LEGION

By the time Justin Minyard discovered the video of himself stoned, drooling and unable to help his daughter unwrap her Christmas presents, he was taking enough OxyContin®, oxycodone and Valium every day to deaden the pain of several terminally ill cancer patients.

"Heroin addicts call it the nod," the former Special Forces soldier says of his demeanor in that video. "My head went back. My eyes rolled back in my head. I started drooling on myself. My daughter was asking why I wasn't helping her, why I wasn't listening to her."

Seeing that video jolted Minyard out of a two-year opiate stupor. He asked a Fort Bragg pain specialist to help him get off the painkillers his primary care physician had prescribed. "I was extremely disappointed in myself," he says. "I knew I couldn't do that to my family again."[1]

The preceding story is just one of many recent anecdotal accounts of veterans struggling with over-prescription of medications. In the best cases, the veteran in question has been able to pull themselves back from the brink, regroup, and work toward a different mode of care that doesn't have the same devastating effect on the veteran and their families. In the worst cases, veterans have died from accidental overdose, or attempted suicide in a medication-induced haze.

In September 2013, CBS news reported the tragic tale of 35 year old Army SPC Scott McDonald, who tragically perished from the accidental overdose brought about by the cumulative effects of the lengthy list of medications he had been prescribed.[2] The American Legion believes these risks increase the importance of exploring Complementary and Alternative Medicine (CAM) therapies[3] that can reduce the over-reliance on prescription drugs and help bring these veterans back from the brink of the abyss.

The American Legion has continued to be concerned with the unprecedented numbers of veterans returning from the wars in Iraq and Afghanistan suffering from TBI and PTSD, categorized as the "signature wounds" of these conflicts. The American Legion believes that all possibilities should be explored and considered in an attempt to finding treatments, therapies, and cures for TBI and PTSD to include alternative treatments and therapies, and they need to make them accessible to all veterans. If these alternative treatments and therapies are deemed effective they should be made available and integrated into the veterans' current health care model of care.

As a result The American Legion established the TBI and PTSD Committee in 2010 comprised of American Legion Past National Commanders, Commission Chairmen, respected academic figures, and national American Legion staff. The Committee is focused on investigating existing science and procedures as well as alternative methods for treating TBI and PTSD that are not being employed by the Department of Defense (DOD) and VA for the purpose of determining if such alternative treatments are practical and efficacious.

During a three year study the Committee met with leading authorities in the DOD, VA, academia, veterans, private sector mental health experts, and caregivers about treatments and therapies veterans have received or are currently receiving for their TBI and PTSD symptoms. Last year the Committee released their findings and recommendations in a report titled "The War Within." "The War Within" report

---

[1] Excerpt "On the Edge" The American Legion Magazine story by Ken Olsen, April 1, 2014.
[2] http://www.cbsnews.com/news/veterans-dying-from-overmedication/
[3] Resolution #108: Request Congress Provide the Department of Veterans Affairs Adequate Funding for Medical and Prosthetic Research

highlights these treatments and therapies and also identifies findings and recommendations to the DOD and VA.

Some of the critical findings of *The War Within* included:

• Most of the existing research for the last several years has only validated the current treatments that already exist—VA and DOD research is not pushing the boundaries of what can be done with new therapies, merely staying within an environment of self-confirmation bias.

• There seems to be a lack of fast track mechanisms within DOD and VA to employ innovative or novel therapies—a standardized approach to these therapies could help servicemembers and veterans gain access to care that could help them.

• While some VA medical centers (VAMCs) do offer complementary alternative medicine (CAM) therapies, they are not offered in a consistent or uniform manner across all 152 VAMCs nationwide—VA struggles with consistency and needs better guidance.

In addition to those findings, the TBI and PTSD Committee made some recommendations for the way forward:

• Congress needs to provide oversight and funding to DOD and the VA for innovative TBI and PTSD research that is being used successfully in the private sector healthcare systems such as hyperbaric oxygen therapy, virtual reality exposure therapy, and non-pharmacological treatments and therapies.[4]

• Congress needs to increase DOD and the VA research and treatment budgets in order to improve the research, screening, diagnosis, and treatments for TBI and PTSD.

• DOD and VA need to accelerate their research efforts in order to effectively and efficiently diagnose and develop evidence-based TBI and PTSD treatments.

The American Legion's efforts to assess the care and treatments available for veterans suffering from TBI and PTSD are not limited to the efforts of the TBI and PTSD Committee. In 2003, The American Legion established the System Worth Saving Task Force to conduct ongoing, on-site evaluations of the Veterans Health Administration (VHA) medical system. Annually, System Worth Saving visits provide Legionnaires, Congress and the public with an in-depth, boots on the ground view of how veterans are receiving their healthcare across the country.

Over the last several years, the System Worth Saving reports have examined the full spectrum of VHA care, but specifically have noted several things about how VHA delivers on complementary and alternative medicine (CAM) in their facilities.

VA medical centers throughout the VA healthcare system are committed, dedicated, and compassionate about treating veterans with TBI. Many medical centers throughout the country have found successful complementary and alternative methods for the treatment of TBI and PTSD such as hiking, canoeing, nature trips, equine, and music therapy.[5] While some systems like the El Paso VA Healthcare System offer several CAM solutions, such as yoga, guitar lesions, sleep hygiene and other practices, other locations such as the Pittsburgh VA and Roseburg VA Healthcare System are more limited, offering only acupuncture in Pittsburgh, and acupuncture for pain management through the fee basis program in Roseburg.[6]

In addition to the ongoing System Worth Saving Task Force visits, The American Legion is taking the lead for veterans by aggressively pursuing the best possible treatment options for veterans on multiple fronts.

On February 3, 2014, The American Legion launched a TBI and PTSD survey online in order to evaluate the efficacy of the veterans' TBI and PTSD care, treatments, and therapies and to find out if they are receiving and benefiting from CAM treatment offered by the DOD and VA. The survey, conducted in coordination with the Data Recognition Corporation (DRC), Dr. Jeff Greenberg, Ph.D., and the Institute for the Advancement of Military and Veteran Healthcare, was to assist The American Legion to better understand the experiences of veterans who receive care throughout the VA healthcare system.

---

[4] Resolution #108: Request Congress Provide the Department of Veterans Affairs Adequate Funding for Medical and Prosthetic Research
[5] 2011 SWS—"Transition of Care from DOD to VA"
[6] 2014 SWS—"Past, Present and Future of VA Health Care"

William Detweiler, Past National Commander and Chairman of the TBI and PTSD Committee has stated about the survey, ''The American Legion is very concerned by the unprecedented number of veterans who suffer from these two conditions * * * We firmly believe that both VA and DOD need to act aggressively in adopting all effective treatments and cures, including alternatives being used in the private sector, and make them available to our veterans nationwide * * *. By completing this survey, veterans across America will have the opportunity to tell the true story of the types of care and treatments that they are actually receiving for PTSD and TBI. The survey will greatly help The American Legion in its efforts to advise the Administration, Congress, DOD, VA on the best possible care and treatments for these injuries.''

The full survey results will be released and discussed in detail at the upcoming American Legion TBI and PTSD Symposium, June 2014, however two key data points emerged which bear special significance to this testimony.

• Medication appears to be the front line treatment reported by respondents.

• A sizable proportion of respondents reported prescriptions of up to 10 medications for PTSD/TBI across their treatment experience.

Both of these data points should raise concerns about whether veterans are getting the right treatment for these signature wounds of the past decade's wars.

SYMPOSIUM:

On June 24, 2014 in Washington, DC, The American Legion is hosting a TBI and PTSD Symposium entitled *"Advancing Care and Treatment for Veterans with TBI and PTSD."* The symposium aims to discuss the findings and recommendations from the TBI and PTSD veteran's survey, and will hear directly from servicemembers, veterans, and caregivers on their TBI and PTSD experiences, treatments and care. The symposium will also help us determine how the Administration, Congress, DOD and VA are integrating complementary and alternative treatments and therapies into current models of veterans' health care.

CONCLUSION:

After a decade of war, America is still grappling with an evolving understanding of the nature of the wounds of warfare. Veterans must be reassured that the care they receive, whether serving on active duty in the military, or through the VA Healthcare system in their home town, is the best treatment available in the world. To combat the physical and psychological wounds of war, sometimes the old treatments are not going to be the most efficacious.

Just as new understanding about the nature of these wounds emerges, so too must the new understanding about the best way to treat these wounds continue to adapt and evolve. Veterans are fortunate to have access to a healthcare system designed to treat their wounds, but that system must recognize that different treatments will have differing levels of effectiveness depending on the individual needs of the wounded veteran. There is no silver bullet. There is no single treatment guaranteed to cure all ailments. With a national policy that respects and encourages alternative therapies and cutting edge medicine, veterans have the best possible shot to get the treatment they need to continue being the productive backbone of society their discipline and training prepares them to be.

Consider the following condensed version of one of the many veteran stories in The American Legion's *The War Within*:

Tim Hecker joined the Army at 18 and soon decided to make a career of it. He served 22 years in all, in and out of combat, rising to the rank of master sergeant. In the summer of 1990, he married his high school sweetheart, Tina, and the couple had three children.

Then Tim couldn't remember having married Tina. He couldn't tell his sons apart. Their names escaped him. Injuries suffered in two separate roadside-bomb explosions in a span of two months in Iraq in early 2008 left him with a Traumatic Brain Injury and severe post-traumatic stress. He was no longer the man Tina had married.

Frustrated with her husband's descent and the lack of progress with traditional care, Tina went online and found information about hyperbaric medicine. Following a phone call and an initial interview, Tim was selected to be part of a pilot study on the use of hyperbaric oxygen therapy (HBOT) for Traumatic Brain Injury (TBI) and Posttraumatic Stress Disorder (PTSD). He claims the treatments have given him back most of his pre-injury life.

> "By the fourth treatment, I started feeling like a new person," he says at his home in West Edmeston, N.Y. "I was more aware. I could see things. The deeper I got into the treatments, my cognition started to come back—my motor skills and my balance. My vision started to improve. The biggest benefit was my emotional control."
>
> "We're talking a 180-degree turn around," Tina says. "There are days when he's almost back to normal with his personality."[7]

Ultimately, that is why it's so important to ensure VA solves the over medication puzzle. The veterans have already returned home from war. This is about helping the veterans to finally return home to their families.

The American Legion looks forward to working with the Committee, as well as VA, to find solutions that work for America's veterans. For additional information regarding this testimony, please contact Mr. Ian de Planque at The American Legion's Legislative Division, (202) 861–2700 or ideplanque@legion.org.

PREPARED STATEMENT OF JOY J. ILEM, DEPUTY NATIONAL LEGISLATIVE DIRECTOR, DISABLED AMERICAN VETERANS

Chairman Sanders, Ranking Member Burr and Members of the Committee: DAV (Disabled American Veterans), an organization of 1.2 million wartime veterans who were wounded, injured or made ill due to their military service, appreciates this opportunity to offer testimony for the record of your hearing to examine overmedication and its problems and solutions in the Department of Veterans Affairs (VA).

Less than a month ago, VA formally directed its 21 Veterans Integrated Service Networks (VISN) to launch a new and intensive opioid safety initiative. The stated goals are to reduce harm to veterans from unsafe medications and dosages, but to adequately control veterans' pain. While DAV offers no opposition to this initiative, our experience in recent years in several local instances with VA physicians who decided to abruptly discontinue prescribed opioids for our members without offering them alternatives does not lend confidence that this initiative will be carried out with sensitivity to the needs of veterans to tolerably manage their pain in absence of such drugs. Some of our members who contacted DAV had been prescribed these drugs for decades, and were tolerating their pain well, but were offered little to no alternatives when VA physicians decided to abruptly end such prescribing. In situations such as these, we are concerned that these veterans will turn to alcohol or illicit drugs in search of pain relief, or will be left to needlessly suffer.

As we understand it, VA's opioid safety initiative contains nine goals. The initial goals (to be accomplished within six months, according to the directive) would establish systems to educate VA prescribers about safely and effectively prescribing opioids; increase the usage of urinalysis to detect presence of opioids in veterans' urine; provide VA prescribers potential access to state prescription databases to identify veterans who are in receipt of opioids from private prescribers; and establish "tapering programs" for certain veterans using opioids along with other drugs.

The second set of VA goals, to be achieved over the next nine months, includes central development of a "risk stratification toolkit" to be deployed locally in VA facilities to enable physicians to assess veterans using opioids who should not be treated with them, or identify those who can be given reduced doses at a safer level. Another goal calls for each VISN to implement a uniform tapering program for certain "high-risk" opioids, with an overall objective of VA's achieving a 75 percent reduction in the use of certain opioids by not later than December 15, 2014.

The third set of VA goals, to be achieved over a year or possibly longer, requires all VA facilities to identify veterans who are prescribed opioids above a stated dosage ceiling (200 milligrams of morphine equivalents per day). VA Central Office will collate this data and provide it to VISNs and facilities, which will be required to conduct appropriateness reviews with prescribers who are identified as providing veterans dosages higher than the dosage ceiling. Another goal is for all VA facilities to provide at least two unspecified complementary and alternative medicine (CAM) modalities in the treatment of chronic pain. These modalities are to be put in place by March 15, 2015.

The last goal is to establish a mental health component within the Patient Aligned Care Team approach to delivering VA care to veterans with a history of prescribed opioid use, focusing on establishing a three-facility trial of deploying "interdisciplinary medication risk management teams," to identify "strong practices that

[7] http://www.legion.org/publications/217301/war-within-treatment-traumatic-brain-injury-and-post-traumatic-stress-disorder

can be operationalized across the VHA Healthcare System,'' to achieve further reductions in the use of prescribed opioids.

The above description of VA's initiative is oversimplified and summarized for the Committee's use, but constitutes our understanding of its purpose based on our review of the directive and information we have received from VA practitioners who remain concerned about this new program's effectiveness and its impact on veterans in pain. To our knowledge neither DAV nor the remainder of the veterans service organization community have had a comprehensive briefing by VA on this new program, its purpose and justification, and how it will be implemented and monitored. It is also our understanding that, although already issued to VISNs and facilities, the directive is being reconsidered based on numerous concerns that have arisen since, and may be amended.

While we have not received a national resolution from our membership on the topic of opioid reduction in VA health care, as indicated above, many of our members who were wounded, injured or made ill due to military service during wartime suffer from chronic pain from numerous causes other than malignancy (the only stated exception to this initiative), and presumably will be targeted by this new policy. The directive suggests that the use of CAM combined with integration of a specialized, and as yet untested, new mental health treatment model can substitute for existing prescribing practices by VA physicians who are dealing over time in primary and specialty care with veterans suffering from chronic pain and chronic pain syndrome.

In a confounding countertrend, the Veterans Benefits Administration recently announced in the *Federal Register* that it has determined justification is sufficient to award service-connected ratings to veterans suffering from chronic pain and chronic pain syndrome, as discrete disabilities. DAV fully supports this broader authority to recognize that chronic pain is real, damaging and even debilitating. Also, this decision on rating veterans with chronic pain would suggest that chronic pain is a significant disabling condition from the vantage point of the VA division that awards disability compensation, whereas based on this new opioid reduction directive, another division of VA may see it quite differently.

DAV is also concerned about VA's potential participation in state drug monitoring programs. Many of these activities were stimulated by law enforcement, not public health authorities, in a search for illicit prescribing practices by private physicians, and trafficking in controlled substances by people who defraud physicians. While we appreciate VA's legitimate interest in protecting against abuse and overuse of opioids, we are concerned about potential unintended consequences of VA's approach to these state monitoring programs and recommend close oversight by the Committee to ensure its purposes are limited to the health and safety of veterans and of their health care.

DAV would never advocate for broad use of narcotics as a first line, or only line, of treatment for wounded, injured and ill veterans with chronic pain or chronic pain syndrome; however, the intent of VA's new initiative seems dedicated first to a drastic reduction in the use of painkiller drugs over other purposes, and may not keep uppermost the needs of veterans who suffer from chronic pain as a clinically legitimate treatment population.

DAV strongly supports bringing significant CAM treatments into VA health care, particularly for younger veterans who do not want traditional health care, prescription medications or typical mental health treatments; however, if VA intends to use CAM as a substitute for, or replacement of, legally prescribed opioid medications in a known and older population, we urge VA to ensure the effects of shifting veterans away from these medications is closely followed in clinical care, lest these veterans resort to the abuse of alcohol or other drugs to compensate for the loss of painkillers that actually work for them. Additionally, VA facilities' selection of CAM models may not have the desired effect intended by this directive. For example, a study in the Journal of the American Medical Association (''Acupuncture for the Treatment of Cocaine Addiction: A Randomized Controlled Trial,'' January 27, 2010) that followed treatment of a large group of cocaine users diverted to acupuncture therapy as a substitute did not demonstrate effectiveness in reducing the use of cocaine in that population. In fact, the study ''does not support the use of acupuncture as a stand-alone treatment for cocaine addiction or in contexts in which patients receive only minimal concurrent psychosocial treatment.'' Numerous other published studies replicate this finding on acupuncture, and are reported on VA's Health Services Research and Development web page, http://www.hsrd.research.va.gov/publications/esp/acupuncture.cfm. In our view, VA health care officials should carefully study the efficacy of CAM modalities as exchanges for prescribed opioids for pain to ensure they can accomplish the results intended, and that CAM modalities selected by facilities are efficacious for these purposes, are evidence-based, and are accompanied by appropriate other treatment resources.

Mr. Chairman, perhaps most important to the purposes of this hearing, DAV is concerned that the required rapid implementation of this new directive will not be standardized and uniform across the vast VA system. In fact, the directive itself allows for local deviations and modifications, by "providing opportunity for customization to meet local needs." The alternative approaches that are offered in the directive are vague, and may lead to wide variations, or only limited local implementation. In DAV's view, the directive should mandate interdisciplinary pain management teams be established at each facility, and ensure these teams are functional, before launching such an aggressive tapering program. The structure and function of such teams should be specified and mandatory. Without more specificity, a "pain management team" may simply become a single provider designated in a facility whose primary (or imposed) clinical role would be to reduce the prescribing of opiates to veterans, without providing viable alternatives to address their pain.

We believe any alternative treatments accompanying this plan should be specified and required in the directive. This availability should include psychological pain management treatments and other alternative treatments, including but not limited to specialized counseling, chiropractic care, and CAM approaches that are evidence-based. Even when some of these services are made "available," a veteran with chronic pain may only be given a limited course of treatment, or be made to choose one or the other but not both to meet pain care needs. This would be an unfortunate and unsafe way to deal with opioid reduction due to its impact on the health of individual veterans. As an advocate for these veterans, especially those who were wounded, injured and ill due to military service, such an outcome would be unacceptable.

During VA's initiative to implement a national formulary 15 years ago, many prescribers complained that they were disallowed from prescribing preferred, standard medications they had used for years in their practices because they were not a part of the then-new national formulary. In order for VA physicians to procure off-formulary drugs under the policy, VA established a national procedure in which the prescriber had to submit an explicit justification for use of a particular drug in an individual veteran's case, before a local or VISN VA pharmacy prescribing board, to gain approval of the deviation. This process at the time was seen as time consuming, a dampening influence, an interference of professional practice, and a difficult bureaucratic barrier. The formulary change accomplished the VA's goal of producing cost savings, but it came at the expense of many veterans who needed to adjust to new medications without warning and in some cases against the interests of their prescribing physicians. We hope and trust this new initiative will not carry similar consequences for the veterans it is going to affect.

Finally, also about 15 years ago, it is helpful to recall that VA took the national and even international lead on establishing pain as the "fifth vital sign." Hospitals and physician practices all over the world now use this concept in evaluating patients' pain level and developing interventions for pain as an important treatment goal on its own merit. Pain is the number one reason people, including wounded, injured and ill veterans, seek health care. DAV hopes VA will be able to carry out this new initiative to reduce opioid prescribing recalling its stewardship of pain management in western medicine, without rushing to judgment that veterans under VA care are atypically overprescribed narcotic medications. We understand from practitioners in VA facilities that, already, the pressure on, and monitoring of, providers to decrease their prescribing of opioids in pain management is leading to significant reductions in such prescribing, with no good alternatives available for affected veterans who are suffering from chronic pain. This is a troubling development, and we hope the Committee will thoroughly review this situation, not only during this hearing but on a recurring basis, to ensure that veterans experiencing pain remain VA's primary focus.

Mr. Chairman and Members, this concludes DAV's statement. Again, DAV appreciates the indulgence of the Committee in permitting the submission of this testimony.

115

PREPARED STATEMENT OF JACQUELINE A. MAFFUCCI, PH.D.,[1] RESEARCH DIRECTOR, IRAQ & AFGHANISTAN VETERANS OF AMERICA

Chairman Sanders, Ranking Member Burr, and Distinguished Members of the Committee: On behalf of Iraq and Afghanistan Veterans of America (IAVA), I would like to extend our gratitude for being given the opportunity to share with you our views and recommendations regarding overmedication, an important issue that affects the lives of thousands of servicemembers and veterans.

As the Nation's first and largest nonprofit, nonpartisan organization for veterans of the wars in Iraq and Afghanistan, IAVA's mission is critically important but simple—to improve the lives of Iraq and Afghanistan veterans and their families. With a steadily growing base of nearly 270,000 members and supporters, we aim to help create a society that honors and supports veterans of all generations.

In partnership with other military and veteran service organizations, IAVA has worked tirelessly to see that veterans' and servicemembers' health concerns are comprehensively addressed by the Department of Veterans Affairs (VA) and by the Department of Defense (DOD). IAVA understands the necessity of integrated, effective, world-class healthcare for servicemembers and veterans, and we will continue to advocate for the development of increased awareness, recognition and treatment of service-connected health concerns.

A recent report from the Center for Investigative Reporting found that over the last 12 years, there has been a 270 percent increase in Veterans Health Administration (VHA) prescriptions for four powerful opiates.[2] There has also been an increase in psychiatric medication prescriptions as well.[3]

Given the last 12 years of conflict and the very physical and psychological demands on our troops, it is no surprise that veterans are seeking care at the VA for a multitude of needs. The use of medication to treat certain physical and mental conditions is a valid treatment option, but the VA must continue to develop a comprehensive and multidisciplinary approach to treatment.

The need for comprehensive treatment is particularly prevalent in polytrauma cases, which are among the most complex medical cases to address. Pain often presents in consort with other conditions, such as depression, anxiety, PTSD, or TBI. Providers can be challenged to treat such polytrauma cases because of the challenge of managing multiple conditions. Some of these conditions may limit the drugs available to the patient, making treatment options limited.

These issues constitute major challenges for providers. Certainly part of a treatment program for chronic pain or mental health issues may include strong medication, including opioids and psychiatric medications; but a schedule of treatment should not be limited to pharmaceutical treatment and should integrate a host of other proven therapies. This is why a stepped case management system can be very helpful. In this type of system, a primary care physician has the support of an integrated, multi-disciplinary team of providers to design and implement a comprehensive treatment plan for the patient.

With approximately 22 veterans dying by suicide every day, and more attempting suicide,[4] reducing instances of overmedication and limiting access to powerful prescription medications that can be used to intentionally overdose must be included in a comprehensive approach to addressing the issue. Particularly considering that overdosing is a common mechanism for suicide attempts, with over half of all nonfatal suicide events among veterans resulting from overdose or intentional poisoning.[5]

The VA's 2012 Suicide Data Report also showed that between 74–80 percent of servicemembers and veterans sought care from a provider within four weeks of attempting suicide.[6] This evidence shows the critical need for providers to not only provide access to timely mental health services, but also to ensure that the risk of

[1] Dr. Jackie Maffucci, IAVA's Research Director, holds a Ph.D. in neuroscience from the University of Texas at Austin. She previously worked with the Provost Marshall General and other senior leaders at the Armed Forces Services Corporation to develop, implement, and monitor research programs and opportunities to address the health and wellness needs of servicemembers.
[2] Glantz, A. (2013, September 28). VA's opiate overload feeds veterans' addictions, overdose death. Center for Investigative Reporting. Retrieved from http://cironline.org/node/5261
[3] Government Accountability Office. (2012, November 14). DOD and VA Healthcare: Medication Needs during Transitions May Not Be Managed for All Servicemembers. Retrieved from http://www.gao.gov/products/GAO–13–26
[4] Kemp, J. and Bossarte, R. (2012). Suicide Data Report 2012. Department of Veterans Affairs. Retrieved from http://www.va.gov/opa/docs/suicide-data-report–2012-final.pdf
[5] Ibid.
[6] Ibid.

overdose and overmedication are minimized through the use of state prescription monitoring programs and the creation of formulary take-back programs.

Given the challenging nature of understanding the medical and mental health needs of veterans, the VA and the DOD have made laudable initiatives to meet these needs. But the challenge remains to uniformly and effectively translate all of these efforts to practice. Too often we hear the stories of veterans who are prescribed what seems like an assortment of psychiatric medications and/or opioids with very little oversight or follow-up. On the flip side, there are also stories of veterans with enormous pain and doctors who won't consider their requests for stronger medication to manage the pain.

One IAVA family member has expressed frustration and concern in regards to the VA's current opioid drug usage. Her husband, who was prescribed nine different medications to address a range of health issues related to pain, anxiety, and depression, tragically passed away from what was labeled an accidental overdose by the corner. Since then, his widow has been fighting for overmedication by the VA to be included on his death certificate.

In a similar case highlighted by CBS, a veteran with 5 tours of duty in Iraq and Afghanistan received a treatment plan from the VA with a total of eight prescriptions. When he was prescribed a ninth drug by the VA he took the medicine as instructed. The next morning he was found by his wife. His death was classified as an accidental death due to overmedication. His widow plans to sue the VA for his death.

It is not our job to second-guess the judgment of the doctors treating these patients, but it is our job to question the system that is providing overall care to our veterans and tracking this care. The VA has established practices and policies aimed at providing quality care to veterans, but it won't do our veterans any good if VHA cannot efficiently and effectively integrate these findings into their management practices and have a plan in place to continually improve upon accepted practice with evidence-based findings. While the VA has made great strides to recognize the need for comprehensive and multidisciplinary support, clearly there is still a lot of room for improvement in implementing these procedures.

In part, some of the challenges may be in the inherent differences between the VA and DOD systems of care, whether it be in their available formularies, uniformity of record keeping and medical terminology used, or the interoperability, or lack thereof, of the medical record systems, care for our military and veteran population should be one integrated approach. A comprehensive treatment plan requires the VA and DOD have an integration of medical records such that receiving doctors are clear on the history of the patients that they intake. But beyond that, once the veteran is received into the VHA system, it's not just about putting out policies, clinical practice guidelines, and funding research. At the end of the day, the success will be seen in how those products are implemented into practice and how they are continually assessed for effectiveness. The key will be in education, integration, and assessment.

Again, we appreciate the opportunity to offer our views on this important topic, and we look forward to continuing to work with each of you, your staff, and this Committee to improve the lives of veterans and their families.

Thank you for your time and attention.

A REPORT BY CITIZENS COMMISSION ON HUMAN RIGHTS INTERNATIONAL
APRIL 2014

A REVIEW OF HOW PRESCRIBED PSYCHIATRIC MEDICATIONS COULD BE DRIVING MEMBERS OF THE ARMED FORCES AND VETS TO ACTS OF VIOLENCE & SUICIDE

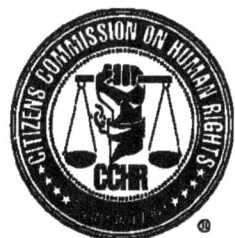

A Report by
Citizens Commission on Human Rights International
April 2014

TABLE OF CONTENTS

INTRODUCTION

The recent tragedies at Fort Hood and the Washington, D.C. Navy Yard are deeply concerning because of the increasing reports of military and veteran violence and suicide in our Armed Forces. Though there can be many reasons for killing oneself or others, the possible role of psychiatric drugs in these tragedies has not been effectively explored. It would be a serious mistake to ignore this factor.

2005 - 2011:

MILITARY PRESCRIPTIONS FOR PSYCHOACTIVE DRUGS INCREASES ALMOST 700 PERCENT.

- Researchers have identified 25 psychiatric medications disproportionately associated with violence, including physical assault and homicide.[1]

- There are 22 international drug-regulatory agency warnings about these medications causing violent behavior, mania, psychosis and homicidal ideation.

- There are almost 50 international drug-regulatory agency warnings about psychiatric drugs causing suicidal ideation.

THERE ARE ABOUT 50 INTERNATIONAL DRUG REGULATORY WARNINGS ABOUT PSYCHIATRIC DRUGS CASUSING SUICIDAL IDEATION.

- One in six American service members were taking at least one psychiatric medication in 2010.[2] More than 110,000 Army personnel were given antidepressants, narcotics, sedatives, antipsychotics and anti-anxiety drugs while on duty in 2011.[3]

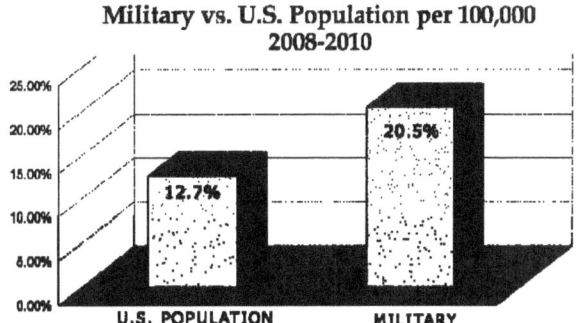

Military vs. U.S. Population per 100,000 2008-2010

U.S. POPULATION: 12.7%
MILITARY: 20.5%

- Between 2005 and 2011 the military increased its prescriptions of psychoactive drugs (antipsychotics, sedatives, stimulants and mood stabilizers) by almost 700 percent, according to *The New York Times*.[4]

- Prescriptions written for antipsychotic drugs for active-duty troops increased 1,083 percent from 2005 to 2011, while the number of antipsychotic drug prescriptions in the civilian population increased just 22 percent.[5]

- The Department of Defense Suicide Event Reports (DoDSERs) for 2012 reported that the Armed Forces Medical Examiner System (AFMES) found that as of 31 March 2013, there were 319 suicides among Active component Service members and 203 among Reserve component Services members. 92.8 percent of the Service Members were male, with 39.6 percent aged between 17 and 24.

ONE IN SIX SERVICE MEMBERS WERE TAKING A PSYCHOACTIVE DRUG IN 2010. RESEARCHERS IDENTIFIED 25 PSYCHIATRIC DRUGS AS PROPORTIONATELY ASSOCIATED WITH VIOLENCE.

- DoDSERs were only included in this report if they were submitted by April 1, 2013 and thus there are discrepancies between the figures reported by the AFMES and the number of DoDSERs included in the DoDSER 2012 report. In addition, there were some DoDSERs that were submitted for events that were still pending a final determination as a suicide.

- A total of 841 Service members had one or more attempted suicides reported in the DoDSER program for CY 2012.

- Some 134 suicide DoDSERs (42.1 percent) and 452 suicide attempt DoDSERs (52 percent) indicated a history of a behavioral disorder.

- The reports also indicated that "93 decedents (29.2 percent) were reported to have ever taken psychotropic[i] medications. A total of 63 decedents (19.8 percent) were known to have used psychotropic medications within 90 days prior to suicide." However, this is likely to be much higher as almost 21 percent of both the "Ever Taken Psychotropic Medication" and the "Use of Psychotropic Medication last 90 days" questions were answered with "Data Unavailable." Potentially up to 50 percent of those committing suicide had at some point taken psychiatric drugs and up to nearly 46 percent had taken them within 90 days.[6]

- The majority (55 percent) of service members who died by suicide during 2008-2010 had never deployed and 84 percent had no documented combat experiences.[7] In the 2012 DoD Suicide Event report on suicide, 52.2 percent of completed suicides had not been deployed in the recent wars and 56.5 percent of suicide attempts had no reported history of deployment.[8]

- The suicide rate increased by more than 150 percent in the Army and more than 50 percent in the Marine Corps between 2001 to 2009.[9] From 2008 to 2010, military suicides were nearly double the number of suicides for the general U.S. population, with the military averaging 20.49 suicides per 100,000 people, compared to a general rate of 12.07 suicides per 100,000 people.[10]

- There are hundreds of "sudden deaths" among veterans that have been prescribed massive cocktails of psychotropic[1] drugs, which a leading neurologist says are "probable sudden cardiac deaths." Yet the practice of prescribing seven or more drugs documented to cause cardiac problems, stroke, violent behavior and suicide (to name but a few of the adverse effects) is still prevalent.

PSYCHOTROPIC MEDICATIONS: ACTS OF VIOLENCE

- FORT HOOD GUNMAN IVAN LOPEZ, 34, was taking Ambien, a sleep agent, and other psychiatric drugs for depression and anxiety when he shot dead three colleagues and injured 16 others before killing himself on April 2, 2014.[11]

- WASHINGTON NAVY YARD SHOOTER AARON ALEXIS, 34, had been prescribed Trazodone killed 12 people and wounded 8, before being killed by police on Sept. 16, 2013.[12]

- SOLDIER PFC. DAVID LAWRENCE, 20, and MARINE LANCE CPL. DELANO HOLMES were both taking Trazodone and other psychiatric medications when they killed a Taliban commander in his prison cell and an Iraqi soldier respectively.[13]

---

[1] *Psychotropic: A term coined in the late 1940s by Ralph Waldo Gerard, an American behavioral scientist and physiologist to medically describe medication capable of affecting the mind, emotions, and behavior—from the Greek, "mind-turning."*

RECOMMENDATIONS

We call for:

1. An inquiry into the potential violence- and suicide-inducing effects of prescribed psychiatric drugs.

2. An investigation into the sudden deaths of vets prescribed cocktails of antipsychotics and other mental health medications with accountability for the deaths and the standard of care given these vets.

3. Full transparency and accountability for the efficacy and results of existing mental health programs for the Armed Forces and veterans.

4. Improved informed consent laws with full searching medical examinations performed before a member of the Armed Forces or veteran can be diagnosed with a mental disorder.

SUPPORTING INFORMATION

PSYCHOTROPIC MEDICATIONS: VIOLENCE RISKS

- It is important to understand that the mental health system for our Armed Forces and veterans often involves the use of psychotropic and neuroleptic[2] drugs. Between 2001 and 2009, orders for psychiatric drugs for the military increased seven fold.[14] In 2010, the *Army Times* reported that one in six service members were taking some form of psychiatric drug.[15]

- A National Institutes of Health website warns consumers to report if while taking Trazodone—one of the drugs prescribed the Navy Yard shooter—they are "thinking about harming or killing yourself," experience "extreme worry; agitation; panic attacks...aggressive behavior; irritability; acting without thinking; severe restlessness; and frenzied abnormal excitement...."[16]

- Psychologists have blamed the surge in random acts of violence among U.S. military on the heavy use of prescribed drugs. "We have never medicated our troops to the extent we are doing now ...And I don't believe the current increase in suicides and homicides in the military is a coincidence," states Bart Billings, a former military psychologist and combat stress expert.[17]

> **"WE HAVE NEVER MEDICATED OUR TROOPS TO THE EXTENT WE ARE DOING NOW... THE CURRENT INCREASE IN SUICIDES AND HOMICIDES IS NO COINCIDENCE."**
>
> **-DR. BART BILLINGS FMR. COL. & ARMY PSYCHOLOGIST**

- The Food and Drug Administration (FDA) MedWatch system that collects adverse drug reports revealed that between 2004 and 2012, there were 14,773 reports of psychiatric drugs causing violent side effects including: 1,531 (10.4 percent) reports of homicidal ideation/homicide, 3,287 (22.3 percent) reports of mania and 8,219 (55.6 percent) reports of aggression.

- Dr. David Healy, a psychiatrist and a former secretary of the British Association for Psychopharmacology estimates that 90 percent of school shooters were users of antidepressants.[18] These same medications are prescribed to at least 6 percent of our servicemen and women.[19]

---

[2] *Neuroleptic: A term coined in 1955 by French psychiatrists Pierre Deniker and Jean Delay to describe the "nerve seizing" effects of major tranquilizers (antipsychotics).*

- *Scientific American* recently reported on a study of the antidepressants paroxetine (Paxil) and fluoxetine (Prozac) involving more than 25,000 subjects, which showed that one out of every 250 were involved in "a violent episode," including 31 assaults and one homicide.[20]

- *Scientific American* also reported the results of a study of more than 9,000 subjects taking paroxetine for depression and other disorders, which found that subjects experienced more than twice as many "hostility events" as subjects taking a placebo.[21]

School Shooters on Antidepressants

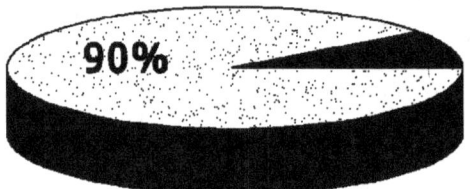

An estimated 90% of school shooters were users of antidepressants, according to Dr. David Healy, psychiatrist.

FDA Medwatch Adverse Psychiatric Drug Reports: 2004-2012

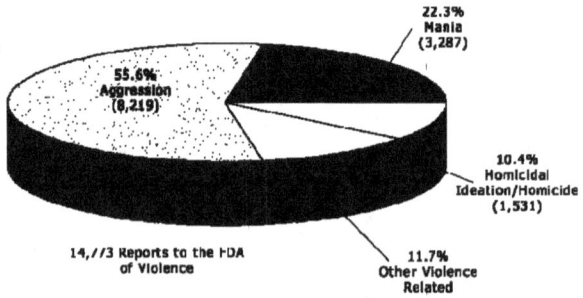

PSYCHOTROPIC MEDICATIONS: SUICIDE

- Between 2005 and 2011, orders for psychiatric drugs for the military increased seven fold.[22]

- Antidepressants carry an FDA "black-box" warning of "suicidality" for those younger than 25. They also have documented side effects of hostility, anxiety and unusual behavior changes for any age group.[23]

- The age range of 41 percent of deployed American soldiers is 18-24 and some are prescribed antidepressants despite the Black Box warning.

- There were 1,304 active and reserve components of the military aged 24 and younger that committed suicide between 1998 and 2011, representing 43.6 percent of 2,990 suicides in this group.[24] The 2012 DoD Suicide Event report found 39.6 percent of the Service members committing suicide were aged 17-24.[25]

  - **A SOLDIER COMMITS SUICIDE EVERY DAY (2013)**

- During 1998-2011 (with the numbers increasing sharply since 2005), 2,990 service members died by suicide while on active duty. Numbers and rates of suicide were highest among service members who were male, in the Army, in their 20s and of white race/ethnicity.[26]

  - **AN ACTIVE-DUTY, RESERVE OR NATIONAL GUARD MEMBER COMMITS SUICIDE EVER 17 HOURS (2012)**

  - **THERE ARE 22 VET SUICIDES EVERY DAY (2010)**

- There was an eightfold increase in martial psychotropic drug use since 2005, with nearly 8 percent of servicemen and women on sedatives and 6 percent on antidepressants.[27]

- In March 2013, the Pentagon reported more soldiers were dying overseas by committing suicide than from combat wounds —about one a day. Returning vets were committing suicide at a rate of 22 each day in 2010—one every 65 minutes.[28]

- In 2012, there was one suicide every 17 hours among all active-duty, reserve and National Guard members, according to figures gathered from each branch.[29]

- The suicide rate increased by more than 150 percent in the Army and more than 50 percent in the Marine Corps between 2001 and 2009.[30]

- The majority (55 percent) of service members who died by suicide during 2008-2010 had never deployed and 84 percent had no documented combat experiences.[31] In the 2012 DoD Suicide Event report on suicide, 52.5 percent of completed suicides had not been deployed in recent wars and 56.5 percent of suicide attempts had no reported history of deployment.[32]

PEOPLE WHO TAKE ANTIDEPRESSANTS "BECOME DISTRAUGHT... THE IRRITABILITY AND IMPULSIVITY CAN MAKE PEOPLE SUICIDAL AND HOMICIDAL."

-DR. JOSEPH GLENMULLEN HARVARD PSYCHIATRIST

- In a report that Health and Human Services and Centers for Medicare and Medicaid Services published in August 2013, it stated, "Antidepressant medications have been shown to increase the risk of suicidal thinking and behavior. In a pooled-analysis of short-term, placebo-controlled trials of nine antidepressant medications, patients taking an antidepressant had twice the risk of suicidality in the first few months of treatment than those taking placebo. The long-term risk is unknown."[33]

Suicides of Active and Reserve Members Aged 24 & Younger

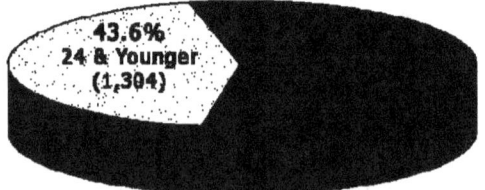

43.6%
24 & Younger
(1,304)

1998 - 2011: 1,304 active and reserve components of the military aged 24 years old and younger committed suicide.

- Harvard Medical School psychiatrist, Dr. Joseph Glenmullen, author of *Prozac Backlash*, says antidepressants could explain the mass-suicides over the last decade. People who take antidepressants, he said, could "become very distraught.... They feel like jumping out of their skin. The irritability and impulsivity can make people suicidal or homicidal."[34]

- Dr. David Healy also determined from a review of published SSRI antidepressant clinical trials that the drugs increase the risk of suicide.[35]

- In February 2005, a study published in the *British Medical Journal* determined that adults taking SSRI antidepressants were more than twice as likely to attempt suicide as patients given placebo.[36]

SUDDEN DEATHS OF SOLDIERS & VETERANS:

The antipsychotic medication Seroquel, referred by vets as "Serokill," is implicated in hundreds of cardiac arrests and sudden deaths of combat veterans.[37]

- In September 2011, the *European Heart Journal* published a study titled, "Psychotropic medications and the risk of sudden cardiac death during an acute coronary event," The researchers concluded: The use of psychotropic drugs, especially combined use of antipsychotic and antidepressant drugs, strongly associated with an increased risk of SCD [sudden cardiac death] at the time of an acute coronary event.[38]

- Dr. Audrey Uy-Evanado reported at the annual meeting of the Heart Rhythm Society in 2013, that both the second-generation and first-generation antipsychotic drugs proved independently associated with greater than threefold increased risks of sudden cardiac deaths.[39]

"THE DEATHS OF THE 'CHARLSTON FOUR' [VETS] WERE PROBABLY CARDIAC DEATHS." ALL "WERE ON THE SAME PRESCRIBED DRUG COCKTAIL" (SEROQUEL, PAXIL, KLONOPIN).

-DR. FRED BAUGHMAN, JR. NEUROLOGIST, HAS LIST OF 395 SUSPECT DEATHS OF SOLDIERS AND VETS.

- California neurologist Dr. Fred Baughman Jr. collected a list of 395 questionable soldier and veteran deaths. He wrote of Andrew White, Eric Layne, Nicholas Endicott and Derek Johnson—all in their twenties, who were West Virginia veterans that died in their sleep in early 2008. "All had been diagnosed 'PTSD'—a psychological diagnosis, not a disease (physical abnormality) of the brain. All were on the same prescribed drug cocktail, Seroquel (antipsychotic), Paxil (antidepressant) and Klonopin (benzodiazepine) and all appeared 'normal' when they went to sleep....the deaths of the 'Charleston Four' were probable sudden cardiac deaths, a sudden, pulseless condition leading to brain death in 4-5 minutes, a survival rate or 3-4 percent, and not allowing time for transfer to a hospital."[40]

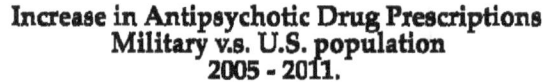

Increase in Antipsychotic Drug Prescriptions Military v.s. U.S. population 2005 - 2011.

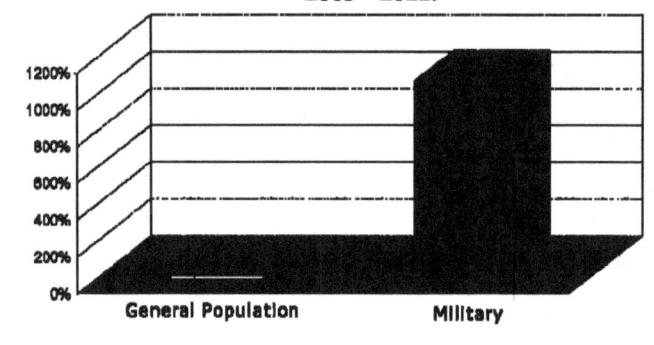

- Sicouri and Antzelevitch (2008) concluded: (1) *"A number of antipsychotic and antidepressant drugs can increase the risk of ventricular arrhythmias and sudden cardiac death," (2) "Antipsychotics can increase cardiac risk even at low doses whereas antidepressants do it generally at high doses or in the setting of drug combinations."*[41]

- The landmark U.S. Clinical Antipsychotic Trials of Intervention Effectiveness (CATIE) study, showed treatment with many atypical antipsychotics is associated with metabolic side effects such as overweight/obesity and diabetes. Failure to properly monitor and manage these effects can lead to increased risk of mortality due to diabetic ketoacidosis [life-threatening problem when the body cannot use sugar as a fuel source because of insufficient or no insulin] and cardiovascular disease.[42]

- Marine Corporal Andrew White, 20, and Senior Airman Anthony Mena, 23, were prescribed a total of 54 drugs between them, including Seroquel, Effexor, Paxil, Prozac, Remeron, Wellbutrin, Xanax, Zoloft, Ativan, Celexa, Cymbalta, Depakote, Haldol, Klonopin, Lexapro, Lithium, Lunesta, Compazine, Desyrel, Trileptal, and Valium, before they died suddenly in their sleep in February 2008 and July of 2009, respectively. The *New York Times* reported, "What killed Airman Mena was not an overdose of any one drug, but the interaction of many."[43]

> **ANTIPSYCHOTIC DRUGS ARE ASSOCIATED WITH GREATER THAN THREE-FOLD INCREASED RISKS OF SUDDEN DEATH.**
>
> -DR. AUDREY UY-EVANDO REPORT TO THE HEART RHYTHM SOCIETY, 2013

- No one is held accountable for prescribing potentially lethal combinations of psychiatric medications to veterans, revealing a discrepancy in the law. Outside the military, doctors have been convicted of manslaughter and culpable negligence for prescribing addictive or dangerous cocktails of medicines. For example, Dr. James Graves' "chemical straightjacket" caused the death of four patients. Florida's Assistant State Attorney Russ Edgar said Graves should have reasonably known his prescriptions were "likely to cause death or great bodily injury."[44] He was sentenced to nearly 63 years in prison.[45]

- A Florida psychiatrist Dr. George Kubski was jailed for one year, given 10-years' probation and ordered to provide $150,000 for a trust fund for the 11-year-old daughter of Jamie Lea Massey, who went to Kubski for pain management and died of drug toxicity. Kubski had prescribed more than 20,000 pills in three months to Mr. Massey.[46]

As stated in the Introduction, prescriptions written for antipsychotic drugs for active-duty troops increased 1,083 percent from 2005 to 2011, while the number of antipsychotic drug prescriptions in the civilian population increased just 22 percent.

Dr. Baughman Jr. points out, "The fact of the matter is that psychotropic drug polypharmacy is never safe, scientific, or medically justifiable."

Further, he called upon "the military for an immediate embargo of all antipsychotics and antidepressants until there has been a complete, wholly public, clarification of the extent and causes of this epidemic of probable sudden cardiac deaths."[47]

POST-TRAUMATIC STRESS DISORDER (PTSD)

The problems for members of the Armed Forces facing war include anguish, fear in battle, sleep deprivation extreme environmental conditions, chemical warfare and vaccines, adding stresses to an already life-threatening environment. Members of the Armed Forces and vets can experience debilitating flashbacks, nightmares and anxiousness.

But to diagnose this as PTSD and imply it is a *physical disease* or *abnormality* is misleading. There is no medical test—no blood or urine test, x-ray or brain scan—that can confirm PTSD is a disease.

• The American Psychiatric Association's *Diagnostic and Statistical Manual of Mental Disorders* (DSM) which lists the symptoms of PTSD has been criticized as unscientific and "clinically risky" which results in the "mislabeling of mental illness in people who will do better without a psychiatric diagnosis," and potentially harmful treatment with psychiatric medication.

• Leading U.S. National Institute of Mental Health-funded researchers of schizophrenia in a 2012 study stated: "The validity of psychiatric diagnosis and the DSM process is the focus of criticism because we have not identified the lesions, the diagnostic process depends upon 'soft' subjective phenomena...."[48]

• A 2013 study in the *Journal of Law, Medicine and Ethics* reported: "It is of no coincidence that this manual (DSM5) relies on a biological disease model of mental illness that is not well supported by the evidence but that does promote the commercial agenda of drug firms...."[49]

- The chairman of the DSM5 Task Force, professor of psychiatry David Kupfer conceded last year that "biological and genetic markers that provide precise [mental health] diagnoses that can be delivered with complete reliability and validity" are still "disappointingly distant."[50]

A chemical imbalance in the brain has been marketed as a "possible" cause of PTSD. Yet even the American Psychiatric Association said that this was a theory that was "probably drug industry derived."[51] It was developed to market antidepressants.

- A study published in 2005 in *PloS Medicine* found that the SSRI antidepressants ads "largely revolved around the claim that SSRIs correct a chemical imbalance caused by a lack of serotonin." Yet, "there is no such thing as a scientifically correct 'balance' of serotonin." Further, "not a single peer-reviewed article ... support[s] claims of serotonin deficiency in any mental disorder," they said.[52]

"THE VALIDITY OF PSYCHIATRIC DIAGNOSIS AND THE DSM PROCESS IS THE FOCUS OF CRITICISM BECAUSE WE HAVE NOT IDENTIFIED THE LESIONS, THE DIAGNOSTIC PROCESS DEPENDS UPON 'SOFT' SUBJECTIVE PHENOMENA...."

- SCHIZOPHRENIA BULLETIN, JANUARY 2012

- In 2013, James Davies, a Senior university Lecturer in Social Anthropology and Psychotherapy said, "despite nearly 50 years of investigation into the theory that chemical imbalances are the cause of psychiatric problems, studies in respected journals have concluded that there is not one piece of convincing evidence the theory is actually correct."[53]

- Yet in 2011, a VA study found that 80 percent of veterans diagnosed with PTSD received psychiatric drugs. Of these, 89 percent were treated with antidepressants, and 34 percent were prescribed antipsychotic drugs.[54]

Members of the Armed Forces and veterans that are told that PTSD is caused by a chemical imbalance in the brain should be informed to require the medical tests to support the diagnosis, otherwise it violates their informed consent rights. One wouldn't undergo chemotherapy without first having the cancer confirmed with tests.

Veterans Diagnosed with PTSD
2011

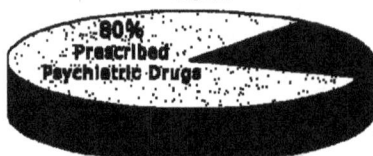

A VA study found 80% of vets diagnosed with PTSD were given psychiatric drugs. Of these, 89% were treated with antidepressants documented to cause suicidal ideation and aggression.

PYCHOTROPIC DRUG USE & COSTS

A 2010 PBS Frontline documentary, *The Wounded Platoon* showed that American soldiers in *combat zones* did not take psychotropic medications prior to the Iraq War, but by the time of the 2007 surge more than 20,000 deployed troops were taking them.[55]

- Veteran Affairs and the Defense Department spent more than $850 million on Seroquel between 2001 and 2011. The antipsychotic is prescribed soldiers to treat "insomnia" for which it is not FDA approved.[56] 1.4 percent of soldiers and 0.7 percent of Marines on active duty in 2010—about 11,000 troops—had received prescriptions for Seroquel.[57]

- Some 54,581 prescriptions for Seroquel were written for active duty service members in 2011 alone—the vast majority as a sleep aid, a condition for which is it not FDA approved to treat.[58]

- Responding to the controversy over Seroquel, in 2012 the DoD conceded that antipsychotics are not an effective treatment for PTSD – a conclusion that an American Medical Association study had reached a year before—and removed Seroquel from its approved formulary list.[59]

- Yet in 2013, the Army announced it was conducting studies on hundreds of vets and service members to evaluate Seroquel and antidepressants to see how the drugs fit into the treatment of traumatized veterans.[60]

- Since 2001, the VA and Defense spent over $790 million on another antipsychotic risperidone.[61] Yet in 2011, the VA reported that Risperdal (risperidone) was no more effective in treating combat stress treatment than a placebo.[62]

- The VA and Defense have spent almost $2 billion to treat mental disorders, which has done nothing to reduce the rate of hospitalization of active troops for these conditions.[63]

- Use of anti-anxiety drugs and sleeping pills such as Valium and Ambien increased 170 percent while spending nearly tripled, from $6 million in 2001 to about $17 million in 2011. Between October 2001 and March 2012, the Defense Department spent a total of $44.1 million on these drugs.[64]

- It spent $2 billion on antipsychotics and anti-anxiety drugs combined over the past decade.

- It also spent at least $2.7 billion on antidepressants.[65]

- In 2012, it was reported the military had spent more than $507 million on Ambien and its generic equivalents.[66] The drug may cause bizarre behavior, hallucinations, abnormal emotions, amnesia, and neuropsychiatric consequences.[67]

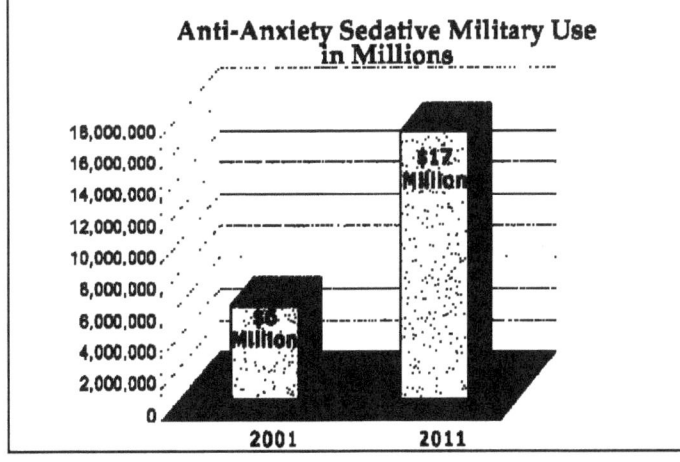

- In 2012, the Army Medical Command warned that the use of benzodiazepines such as Xanax and Valium could intensify combat stress symptoms and lead to addiction.[68] The Army Surgeon General's office also warned regional medical commanders against using anti-anxiety meds such as Klonopin, Ativan and Valium to treat PTSD.[69]

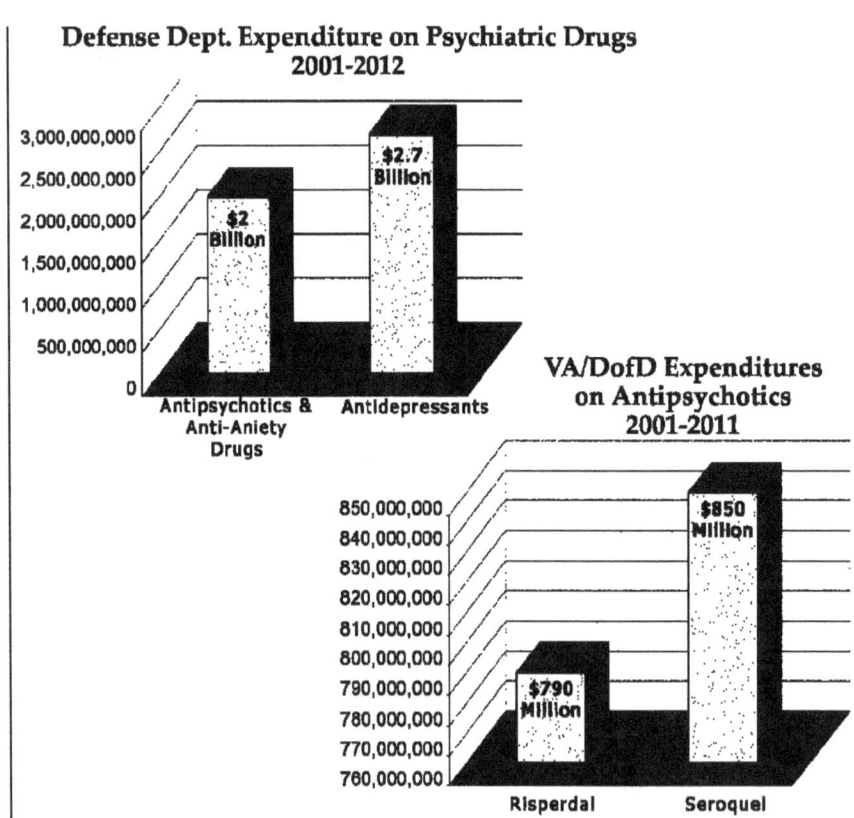

Defense Dept. Expenditure on Psychiatric Drugs 2001-2012

VA/DofD Expenditures on Antipsychotics 2001-2011

Although normally prescribed to treat psychotic disorders, anti-psychotics are largely being prescribed to treat insomnia in the military - for which they are not FDA approved.

LEGAL JUDGMENTS REGARDING PSYCHIATRIC

DRUGS & VIOLENCE

December 2011: Winnipeg, Canada judge Justice Robert Heinrichs ruled that a 15-year-old boy murdered his friend due to the effects of Prozac, stating: "He had become irritable, restless, agitated, aggressive and unclear in his thinking. It was while in state he overreacted in an impulsive, explosive and violent way. Now that his body and mind are free and clear of any effects of Prozac, he is simply not the same youth in behavior and character."[70]

June 2001: A Wyoming jury awarded $8 million to the relatives of a man, Donald Schell, who went on a shooting rampage after taking Paxil and killing his wife, daughter and his granddaughter. Harvard psychiatrist John Maltsberger testified that SSRI manufacturers should warn that antidepressants could cause some patients to experience akathisia and mania, which can induce violent behavior and suicide.[71]

May 25, 2001: An Australian judge blamed the antidepressant Zoloft for turning a peaceful, law-abiding man, David Hawkins, into a violent killer. Judge Barry O'Keefe said that had Mr. Hawkins not taken the antidepressant, "it is overwhelmingly probable that Mrs. Hawkins would not have been killed...."[72] Further, "The killing was totally out of character" and "inconsistent with the loving, caring relationship which existed between him and his wife and with their happy marriage of 50 years."[73]

January 1999: University of North Dakota student Ryan Ehlis, 27, shot and killed his five-week-old daughter and wounded himself after taking the stimulant Adderall for several weeks. Shire Richwood, the manufacturer of Adderall, issued a statement to the court that psychosis is a side effect of this class of stimulants. Charges were dismissed against Ehlis after various doctors testified that he suffered from "Amphetamine-Induced Psychotic Disorder."[74]

INFORMED CONSENT RIGHTS

According to Dr. Baughman, Jr., "In no edition of the DSM are psychiatric diagnoses actual physical abnormalities of the body or brain making them diseases, disorders, or syndromes in a medical sense." All such statements are false, he adds, stating that, therefore, "no such patient has been accorded his or her right on informed consent."

A study of Direct-to-Consumer Advertising of psychotropic drugs pointed out that "None of the advertisements include detailed information on talk therapy or exercise, which have both been proven to help ease the stress of mental conditions—In fact, advertisements often go as far as to claim that 'only your doctor can diagnose depression,' when this simply is not true." This then directs the person to a doctor's office where they're most likely to receive a prescription.

The study cited one ad for the antidepressant Prozac, which stated that "talk therapy cannot control the medical causes of depression."[76]

Alternative approaches to helping the mental health needs of the Armed Forces and veterans can be disregarded in the face of a "quick fix pill," thereby violating informed consent rights. Dr. Hyla Cass, psychiatrist, reported that many drugs, such as the stimulants Ritalin and Adderall can reduce appetite. This, in turn, decreases the intake of beneficial nutrients. Some antidepressants also tend to have this appetite-reducing effect. Many of the neuroleptics (antipsychotic drugs) and some antidepressants cause insulin resistance or metabolic syndrome, with resulting blood sugar swings.[77]

Lt. Col. Charles Ruby, who retired from the Air Force launched Operation Speak Up to help establish group settings for veterans to talk about their combat stress, based on the Alcoholics Anonymous model. "Our view is that psychiatric drugs do nothing but sedate people. We believe that speaking out is a much better way to treat these people and to find a way to integrate back into their communities."[78]

A cost-benefit analysis must be done on existing mental health programs and the impact of these on the mental health of the nation, at the exclusion of alternative methods of help. Informed consent requires that all patients be informed of the subjective nature of a psychiatric diagnosis, the right to refuse to consent to psychiatric medication and the right to know about alternatives available.

CASE EXAMPLES

SGT. VINCINTE JACKSON, 40, stabbed to death Spc. Brandy Fonteneaux, 28, on January 8, 2012. He was convicted of and sentenced to life in prison for the unpremeditated murder and said he was "horrified" by the crime and takes full responsibility for his actions. But he doesn't know why he did it. A defense attorney, Capt. Jeremy Horn, said that a combination of heavy drinking and a prescription antidepressant, Celexa, left Jackson unable to control his own actions or form any kind of plan to commit murder.[79]

MARINE LANCE CPL. DELANO HOLMES, 22, fatally stabbed an Iraqi soldier to death in 2007 after being prescribed Trazodone, Ambien and Valium.[80] He was convicted of negligent homicide and received a bad conduct discharge from the Marines.[81]

FORMER U.S. ARMY SPECIALIST KYLE WESOLOWSKI returned from Iraq in December 2010 following a brutal yearlong deployment. Psychiatrists at Fort Hood gave him "a cocktail of seven different drugs" for war-related mental health issues. More than three years later, Wesolowski came to the uncomfortable conclusion that the prescribed drugs made him homicidal. He contemplated murdering a young woman he met in a bar near the base. "I began to fantasize about killing her," he said. Wesolowski, who is now off of most of the drugs he formerly took, is using his GI Bill benefits to attend college in Thailand.[82]

SPC. ANDREW TROTTO, a 24-year-old Army gunner, was prescribed as many as 20 psychiatric medications, starting while in combat in Iraq when he had difficulty falling asleep. He was prescribed the antipsychotic Seroquel. His body adapted to it and he was soon taking a dose meant for psychotics. "They had no clue what the hell they were doing," Trotto says of the doctors at the battalion aid station who prescribed the pills. "They just throw you on a drug, and if it doesn't work, they throw you on something else. 'Try this. Try this. Try this.'" In addition to Seroquel, he was taking the antidepressant Zoloft and Vicodin to relieve pain from ruptured disks he sustained falling nine feet off a tank. "Let me remind you," he says, "I was a gunner, completely whacked out of my mind. There were quite a few of us on Seroquel and antidepressants." While in a warrior-recovery unit in Kuwait, he locked himself in an outside toilet with a loaded M16 in his mouth, but he managed to hold out long enough to seek help. "I told them, 'You need to do something, or I am going to take other people out with me.'" His mother, Gina, says: "This was the all-American kid. He never had psychiatric problems or problems with suicide. They took a young man who was reacting normally to an abnormal situation – which is war – and they shoved him on an antipsychotic. I watched him become a completely different person. My son ended up gaining 40 pounds from all these medications... I was watching my son slowly die."[83]

RONALD BRUCE WEDDERMAN, 55, a National Guard staff sergeant who fought in Iraq in 2005, returned home and VA doctors prescribed him the antidepressant Trazadone for sleep and Prozac. He says the combination was nearly lethal. "At one point I had two pistols raised to my head on the beach. Somebody called the police. They found me yelling and screaming at people and waving my guns." Wedderman has not taken Trazadone again, and he hasn't tried to kill himself, either.[84]

JOHN KEITH, 35. In a single visit, a VA doctor put him on Seroquel and the antidepressants Trazadone and Zoloft. "I called my doctor up and said, 'I just threw my friend's furniture off a third-story balcony.' [The doctor] said, 'Well, just cut the new pills in half'... At first they give you one or two or three, and you try those for a couple of weeks....But they keep giving you more and more, and by the end of it, you're on 17 medications." Since getting off the drugs and forming an organization to help vets manage their paperwork, Keith has processed more than a thousand veterans' disability claims. He says, "I have never seen a veteran who is or was on less than five medications."[85]

KELLI GRESE: On Veterans Day 2010, former Navy corpsman Kelli, 37, swallowed an unknown quantity of the antipsychotic Seroquel — her fourth suicide attempt in eight months using the same drug. Her death was the subject of a $5 million lawsuit filed against the VA in December 2012.[86] The government ultimately settled the lawsuit, although it admitted no liability.[87] Between 1991 and 1997, Kelli and her sister, Darla served in the U.S. Navy. In 1995, while serving in Naples, Italy, they were the victims of a home invasion by three men. Although they were physically unharmed, they were diagnosed with PTSD. Kelli continued to be a highly functioning, exceptional sailor: Her evaluations were superb; she was nominated for Junior Sailor of the Quarter at the end of her career; she managed and participated on the command color guard team. However, she was discharged from the Navy due to the PTSD and migraine headaches. There followed years of being prescribed up to 20 different psychotropic drugs as well as painkillers. In 1999, according to Darla, who kept meticulous records of Kelli's medication, 5,370 Klonopin, an anti-anxiety drug, were prescribed. Kelli worsened. In 2002, the VA began her on a "trial" of Seroquel in addition to other drugs, including Zoloft and Geodon. She attempted suicide. And still, her medication list ballooned until on November 12, 2010, she killed herself.[88]

CPL. CHAD OLIGSCHLAEGER, 21: For seven months in 2006, the marine patrolled a war-torn city in Iraq. When he returned to his home base he drank heavily, panicked at the sound of a car backfire, swerved around potholes as if they were roadside bombs and had visions of dead friends. He was diagnosed with PTSD and recommended him for a substance abuse clinic in San Diego. Instead, he was sent to a month of live-fire training in a mock Iraqi village in the High Desert in preparation for another deployment. Although the second deployment was less violent, his return to Iraq plunged him into the memories of his first tour. He was recommended psychoactive drugs, starting with Prozac. Over the next two months, Oligschlaeger's symptoms worsened, but his prescriptions increased and by mid-May, he had at least seven active prescriptions, totaling 18 pills a day. He was found dead on the floor of his barracks room on May 20, 2008. All signs pointed to suicide. But an autopsy revealed he had taken the pills that military doctors gave him, dying of accidental "multiple drug toxicity." The Marine's blood held a mix of two antidepressants, an antipsychotic, two kinds of benzodiazepine, and propranolol, a beta blocker sometimes used to subdue fears. A seventh drug was a small amount of methamphetamine, which may have been from illegal drug use or it could be a false positive from over-the-counter medication. None of these drugs had been taken in deadly dosage, but together they had proven fatal.[89]

THE CITIZENS COMMISSION ON HUMAN RIGHTS INTERNATIONAL

The Citizens Commission on Human Rights (CCHR) is a non-profit, non-political and non-religious mental health watchdog established in 1969 by the Church of Scientology and the late Dr. Thomas Szasz, professor of psychiatry, Syracuse University of New York Health Science Center. It works to enact protections for and increase consumer rights especially informed consent rights, and raises public awareness about psychiatric abuses.

It has assisted many thousands of individuals who have been adversely treated in the U.S. mental health system and around the world. It is the only group that has obtained more than 160 consumer/mental health patient-protection laws in the world, receiving recognition from the Special Rapporteur to the United Nations Human Rights Commission for being "responsible for many great reforms."

Several Congressional recognitions of our work includes a Resolution by Congressman Diane Watson, which "highly commends CCHR for securing numerous reforms around the world, safeguarding others from abuses in the mental health system and ensuring legal protections are afforded them."

Its board of advisors, called Commissioners, includes doctors, psychologists, attorneys, educators, artists, businessmen, and civil and human rights representatives.

CCHR's work aligns with the UN Universal Declaration of Human Rights, in particular the following precepts: Article 3: Everyone has the right to life, liberty and security of person and Article 5: "No one shall be subjected to torture or to cruel, inhuman or degrading treatment or punishment."

CCHR International
6616 Sunset Blvd. Los Angeles, California 90028 U.S.A.
Tel: (323) 467-4242
E-mail: humanrights@cchr.org
Website: http://www.cchrint.org

REFERENCES

[1] Thomas J. Moore, Joseph Glenmullen, Curt D. Furbert, "Prescription Drugs Associated with Reports of Violence Towards Others," Public Library of Science ONE, Vol. 5, Iss. 12, Dec. 2010, http://www.plosone.org/article/info%3Adoi%2F10.1371%2Fjournal.pone.0015337.

[2] Andrew Tilghman and Brendan McGarry, "Medicating the military: Use of psychiatric drugs has spiked; concerns surface about suicide, other dangers," Army Times, 17 Mar. 2010, http://www.armytimes.com/article/20100317/NEWS/3170315/Medicating-military

[3] "A fog of drugs and war," The Los Angeles Times, 7 Apr. 2013, http://articles.latimes.com/2012/apr/07/nation/la-na-army-medication-20120408/2.

[4] Richard A. Friedman, "War on Drugs," The New York Times, 6 Apr 2013; http://www.nytimes.com/2013/04/07/opinion/sunday/wars-on-drugs.html?ref=opinion&_r=0&gwh=7E028A441FC225E6745B9904CFDA2A92&gwt=pay

[5] Ibid.

[6] "Department of Defense Suicide Event Report Calendar Year 2012 Annual Report," National Center for Telehealth & Technology (T2), Department of Defense Suicide Event Reports, Generated on 12/20/13 RefID: 7-AF33A11.

[7] "Deaths by Suicide While on Active Duty, Active and Reserve Components, U.S. Armed Forces, 1998-2011," http://timemilitary.files.wordpress.com/2012/07/msmrsuicide2012-06.pdf

[8] "Department of Defense Suicide Event Report Calendar Year 2012 Annual Report," National Center for Telehealth & Technology (T2), Department of Defense Suicide Event Reports, Generated on 12/20/13 RefID: 7-AF33A11.

[9] Martha Rosenberg, "Why Are Suicides Climbing in the Military? Let's Look at the Drugs Being Prescribed," AlterNet, 2 Feb. 2013.

[10] "US Special Ops forces committing suicide in record numbers," RT.com, 19 Apr. 2014, http://rt.com/usa/special-ops-record-suicide-rate-536/

[11] David Montgomery, Manny Fernandez and Timothy Williams, "Fort Hood Gunman Was Being Treated for Depression," The New York Times, 3 Apr 2014, http://www.nytimes.com/2014/04/04/us/fort-hood-shooting.html?_r=0.

[12] Trip Gabriel, Joseph Goldstein and Michael S. Schmidt. "Suspect's Past Fell Just Short of Raising Alarm," The New York Times, 17 Sep 2013.

[13] http://www.presstv.com/detail/2013/09/20/324976/navy-yard-shooter-was-on-trazodone/;http://www.presstv.com/detail/2013/09/20/324976/navy-yard-shooter-was-on-trazodone/; "Lawyers: Marine was being treated [LCp Delano Holmes still in brig, still awaits day in court]" San Diego Tribune, 1 Nov. 2007, http://www.freerepublic.com/focus/f-news/1919611/posts

[14] Op Cit., Andrew Tilghman and Brendan McGarry, "Medicating the military."

[15] Ibid.

[16] http://www.nlm.nih.gov/medlineplus/druginfo/meds/a681038.html

[17] "Prescribed drugs 'to blame over spate of violence among US soldiers'" Daily Telegraph (UK), 9 Apr. 2012, http://www.telegraph.co.uk/news/worldnews/northamerica/usa/9193850/Prescribed-drugs-to-blame-over-spate-of-violence-among-US-soldiers.html; "Soldiers at war in fog of psychotropic drugs," The Seattle Times, 9/10 April 2012, http://seattletimes.nwsource.com/html/nationworld/2017944964_drugsofwar10.html.

[18] "Radical increase in kids prescribed Ritalin," WND, 1 Apr. 2013, http://www.wnd.com/2013/04/radical-increase-in-kids-prescribed-ritalin/#hQjxdxIizztQyRWY.99.

[19] Op Cit.,"A fog of drugs and war," The Los Angeles Times.

[20] John Hogan, "Did Antidepressant Play a Role in Navy Yard Massacre?" Scientific American, 20 Sept. 2013, http://blogs.scientificamerican.com/cross-check/2013/09/20/did-antidepressant-play-a-role-in-navy-yard-massacre/

[21] Ibid.

[22] Op. Cit., Richard A. Friedman, The New York Times.

[23] Op Cit., "Radical increase in kids prescribed Ritalin"

[24] "Deaths by Suicide While on Active Duty, Active and Reserve Components, U.S. Armed Forces, 1998-2011," http://timemilitary.files.wordpress.com/2012/07/msmrsuicide2012-06.pdf

[25] "Department of Defense Suicide Event Report Calendar Year 2012 Annual Report," National Center for Telehealth & Technology (T2), Department of Defense Suicide Event Reports, Generated on 12/20/13 RefID: 7-AF33A11.

[26] "Deaths by suicide while on active duty, active and reserve components, U.S. Armed Forces, 1998-2011,"PubMed.gov, June 2012, http://www.ncbi.nlm.nih.gov/pubmed/22779434

[27] Op Cit., "A fog of drugs and war." The Los Angeles Times.

[28] "Military Suicides Hit Epidemic Levels," American Free Press, 27 Mar. 2013, http://www.huffingtonpost.com/2013/01/14/military-suicides-2012_n_2472895.html

[29] "One every 18 hours: Military suicide rate still high despite hard fight to stem deaths," NBC News. 23 May, 2013, http://usnews.nbcnews.com/_news/2013/05/23/18447439-one-every-18-hours-military-suicide-rate-still-high-despite-hard-fight-to-stem-deaths?lite

[30] Martha Rosenberg, "Why Are Suicides Climbing in the Military? Let's Look at the Drugs Being Prescribed," AlterNet, 2 Feb 2013.

[31] "Deaths by Suicide While on Active Duty, Active and Reserve Components, U.S. Armed Forces, 1998-2011." http://timemilitary.files.wordpress.com/2012/07/msmrsuicide2012-06.pdf

[32] "Department of Defense Suicide Event Report Calendar Year 2012 Annual Report," National Center for Telehealth & Technology (T2), Department of Defense Suicide Event Reports, Generated on 12/20/13 RefID: 7-AF33A11.

[33] "APTYICAL ANTIPSYCHOTIC MEDICTIONS: USE IN ADULTS," Dept. Health and Human Services, Centers for Medicare and Medicaid Services, Aug. 2013, p. 4. http://www.cms.gov/Medicare-Medicaid-Coordination/Fraud-Prevention/Medicaid-Integrity-Education/Pharmacy-Education-Materials/Downloads/atyp-antipsych-adult-factsheet.pdf

[34] "FDA Mulls Antidepressant Warnings," Daily Press, 21 Mar. 2004.

[35] David Healy, Graham Aldred, "Antidepressant drug use & the risk of suicide," International Review of Psychiatry, June 2005, 17 (3), pp.163-172.

[36] "Drug Raise Risk of Suicide; Analysis of Data Adds to Concerns on Antidepressants," The Washington Post, 18 Feb. 2005.

[37] Martha Rosenberg, "Are Veterans Being Given Deadly Cocktails to Treat PTSD?" AlterNet, 6 Mar 2010, http://www.alternet.org/world/145892/are_veterans_being_given_deadly_cocktails_to_treat_ptsd?page=1.

[38] "Psychotropic medications and the risk of sudden cardiac death during an acute coronary event," Eur Heart J first published online September 14, 2011 doi:10.1093/eurheartj/ehr368

[39] "Antipsychotics linked to sudden cardiac death risk," Clinical Psychiatry News, 24 Apr.2013, http://www.clinicalpsychiatrynews.com/cme/click-for-credit-articles/single-article/antipsychotics-linked-to-sudden-cardiac-death-risk/72b732346f34c5553e33532f7ba38914.html

[40] "Psychotropic medications and the risk of sudden cardiac death during an acute coronary event," Eur Heart J first published online September 14, 2011 doi:10.1093/eurheartj/ehr368

[41] Fred A. Baughman, Jr. M.D., Stanley White. "Hundreds of Soldiers & Vets Dying From Antipsychotic—Seroquel," PR Newswire, 7 Nov. 2011, http://www.prnewswire.com/news-releases/hundreds-of-soldiers--vets-dying-from-antipsychotic--seroquel-133366423.html

[42] Richard R Owen et al, "Monitoring and managing metabolic effects of antipsychotics: a cluster randomized trial of an intervention combining evidence-based quality improvement and external facilitation," Implementation Science 2013, 8:120, http://www.implementationscience.com/content/8/1/120; http://www.implementationscience.com/content/pdf/1748-5908-8-120.pdf

[43] "For Some Troops, Powerful Drug Cocktails Have Deadly Results," The New York Times, 12 Feb. 2011, http://www.nytimes.com/2011/02/13/us/13drugs.html?pagewanted=all&_r=0

[44] "Graves guilty: Pace doctor convicted in 4 drug deaths," Pensacola News Journal, 20 Feb., 2002.

[45] "Doctor gets 63 years in OxyContin deaths." Chicago Tribune News, 23 Mar. 2002,

144

[46] "Psychiatrist gets year for patient's pill death," *Palm Beach Post*, 1 Feb. 2003.

[47] "Hundreds of Soldiers & Vets Dying from Antipsychotic—Seroquel," PR Newswire, 7 Nov. 2011.

[48] John M. Kane, Barbara Cornblatt, et al, "Schizophrenia Bulletin," Jan 2012 http://www.ncbi.nlm.nih.gov/pmc/articles/PMC3245590/.

[49] Marc A. Rodwin, J.D., Ph.D., "Institutional Corruption & Pharmaceutical Policy," *Journal of Law, Medicine and Ethics*, 41, No. 3 (2013).

[50] http://www.medscape.com/viewarticle/803752.

[51] Interview of Dr. Mark Graff on *CBS Studio 2*, July 2005.

[52] Jeffrey R. Lacasse and Jonathan Leo, "Depression: A Disconnect between the Advertisements and the Scientific Literature," *Plos Medicine*. Vol 2.e392, Dec. 2005; Sharon Begley, "Some Drugs Work To Treat Depression, But It Isn't Clear How," *The Wall Street Journal*, 18 Nov. 2005.

[53] "Does your child really have a behaviour disorder? A shocking book by a leading therapist reveals how millions of us – including children – are wrongly labeled with psychiatric problems," *The Daily Mail (UK)*, 6 May 2013.

[54] "Pharmacotherapy of PTSD in the U.D. Department of Veterans Affairs: diagnostic- and symptom-guided drug selection," *J Clin Psychiatry*, Jun 2008; 69(6):959-65.

[55] Jamie Reno, "'Medicating Our Troops Into Oblivion': Prescription Drugs Said To Be Endangering U.S. Soldiers," *International Business Times*, 19 Apr. 2014, http://www.ibtimes.com/medicating-our-troops-oblivion-prescription-drugs-said-be-endangering-us-soldiers-1572217

[56] "Seroquel .k.a.'Serokill'",http://ww1.prweb.com/prfiles/2012/12/06/10213863/Seroquel%20or%20Serokill.pdf, citing "VA/Defense Mental Health Drug Expenditures Since 2001," May 2012 Drug Totals, *Government Executive*, http://cdn.govexec.com/media/gbc/docs/pdfs_edit/051712bb1_may2012drugtotals

[57] "Mental Illness is Leading Cause of Hospitalization for Active-Duty Troops," Nextgov., 17 May 2012, http://www.nextgov.com/health/2012/05/mental-illness-leading-cause-active-duty-troops/55797/

[58] Kelley Vlahos, "The Military's Prescription Drug Addiction Overmedication is an epidemic in our armed forces—and claims lives far from the battlefield," *The American Conservative*, 3 Oct. 2013, http://www.theamericanconservative.com/articles/the-militarys-prescription-drug-addiction/

[59] *Op. Cit.*, Jamie Reno, *International Business Times*.

[60] "Military Announces Clinical Trials Set For PTSD Drugs," Pharma Watchdog, 18 Dec. 2013, http://www.pharmawatchdog.com/clinical-trials-ptsd-drugs

[61] http://cdn.govexec.com/media/gbc/docs/pdfs_edit/051712bb1_may2012drugtotals.pdf

[62] *Op Cit.*, Martha Rosenberg, "Are Veterans Being Given Deadly Cocktails to Treat PTSD?"

[63] "Mental Illness is the Leading Cause of Hospitalization of Active-Troops," Nextgov, 17 May, 2012, http://www.nextgov.com/health/2012/05/mental-illness-leading-cause-hospitalization-active-duty-troops/55797/

[64] "Mental Illness is Leading Cause of Hospitalization for Active-Duty Troops." Nextgov., 17 May 2012, http://www.nextgov.com/health/2012/05/mental-illness-leading-cause-hospitalization-active-duty-troops/55797/

[65] *Ibid.*

[66] "Soaring cost of military drugs could hurt budget," Statesman.com, 29 Dec. 2012, http://www.statesman.com/news/news/national-govt-politics/the-soaring-cost-of-military-drugs/nThwF/

[67] N. Gunja, "The clinical and forensic toxicology of Z-drugs," J Med Toxicol. 2013 Jun;9(2):155-62. doi: 10.1007/s13181-013-0292-0; http://www.ncbi.nlm.nih.gov/pubmed/23404347

[68] "Mental Illness is the Leading Cause of Hospitalization of Active Troops," Nextgov, 17 May, 2012, http://www.nextgov.com/health/2012/05/mental-illness-leading-cause-hospitalization-active-duty-troops/55797/

[69] Op. Cit., Jamie Reno, "'Medicating Our Troops Into Oblivion'"

[70] "'Prozac Defence' stands in Manitoba teen's murder case," The National Post (Canada), 11 Dec. 2011.

[71] H. Michael Steinberg, "Colorado Criminal Law - Studies Helpful to Understanding Defense Based Upon Prescription Drug - Medication - Induced Crimes," http://www.colorado-drug-lawyer.com.

[72] Sarah Boseley, "Prozac class drug blamed for killing," The Guardian (London), 2 May 2001.

[73] Jim Rosack, "SSRIs Called on Carpet Over Violence Claims," Psychiatric News, Vol. 36, No. 19, 5 Oct. 2001.

[74] "Prescription: concentration. The number of prescriptions for Adderall is rising, as is the number of students using the drug for academic and recreational purposes," Oregon Daily Emerald, 2 May 2005; "Man who Shot Child Sues Drug Company," Herald, 23 Sept. 2000.

[75] Megan Nugent, Public Justice Department, SUNY Oswego, DTC Advertising of Psychotropic Medications and its Role in the Perception of Mental Illness, http://www.oswego.edu/Documents/wac/Public%20Justice.pdf.

[76] Ibid.

[77] http://www.huffingtonpost.com/hyla-cass-md/is-your-medication-robbin_b_679382.html.

[78] Kelley Beaucar Vlahos, "The Military's Prescription Drug Addiction Overmedication is an epidemic in our armed forces—and claims lives far from the battlefield," The American Conservative, 3 Oct. 2013, http://www.theamericanconservative.com/articles/the-militarys-prescription-drug-addiction/

[79] "Colorado Soldier Guilty Of Unpremeditated Murder," CBS Denver, 13 Dec. 21012, http://denver.cbslocal.com/2012/12/13/colorado-soldier-guilty-of-unpremeditated-murder/; "Army Sergeant Gets Life in Barracks Slaying," Military.com, 14 Dec. 2012, http://www.military.com/daily-news/2012/12/14/army-sergeant-gets-life-in-barracks-slaying.html; Celexa reference http://ssristories.org/expert-testifies-that-pills-alcohol-led-soldier-to-kill-stars-and-stripes/ citing, Jakob Rodgers, The Gazette, 12 Dec, 2012

[80] http://www.presstv.com/detail/2013/09/20/324976/navy-yard-shooter-was-on-trazodone/; "Lawyers: Marine was being treated [LCp Delano Holmes still in brig, still awaits day in court]" San Diego Tribune, 1 Nov. 2007, http://www.freerepublic.com/focus/f-news/1919611/posts

[81] "Critics at war with military justice," Chicago Tribune, 20 Jan. 2008, http://articles.chicagotribune.com/2008-01-20/news/0801190157_1_delano-holmes-iraqi-soldier-military-justice; http://pqasb.pqarchiver.com/indystar/results.html?Title=%22Indy+Marine+won%27t+serve+more+time+for+Iraqi%27s+death%22

[82] Op. Cit., Jamie Reno, "'Medicating Our Troops Into Oblivion.'"

[83] Paul John Scott, "The Military's Billion-Dollar Pill Problem," Men's Journal, Dec. 2012, http://www.mensjournal.com/magazine/the-militarys-billion-dollar-pill-problem-20130116

[84] Ibid.

[85] Ibid.

[86] "Sailor's suicide triggers lawsuit against VA," USA Today, 7 Dec. 2012, http://www.usatoday.com/story/news/nation/2012/12/07/suicide-lawsuit-va/1754705/

[87] Julie Driscoll, "Navy Veteran Kelli Grese: A victim of deadly military drugging," Examiner.com, 2 July 2013, http://www.examiner.com/article/navy-veteran-kelli-grese-a-victim-of-deadly-military-drugging

[88] Ibid.

[89] "PTSD: Battling the shock of war," Navy Times, 25 Mar. 2014, http://www.navytimes.com/article/20140325/NEWS/303250058/PTSD-Battling-shock-war

www.ingramcontent.com/pod-product-compliance
Lightning Source LLC
Chambersburg PA
CBHW080813180526
45168CB00006B/2428

9 7 8 1 5 1 7 7 6 2 1 1 7